History of Medicine

It is sobering to realise that as recently as the year in which On the Origin of Species was published, learned opinion was that diseases such as typhus and cholera were spread by a 'miasma', and suggestions that doctors should wash their hands before examining patients were greeted with mockery by the profession. The Cambridge Library Collection reissues milestone publications in the history of Western medicine as well as studies of other medical traditions. Its coverage ranges from Galen on anatomical procedures to Florence Nightingale's common-sense advice to nurses, and includes early research into genetics and mental health, colonial reports on tropical diseases, documents on public health and military medicine, and publications on spa culture and medicinal plants.

Practical Treatise on the Bath Waters, Tending to Illustrate their Beneficial Effects in Chronic Diseases

Bath physician Joseph Hume Spry (*c.*1779–1859) was concerned that the popular practice of 'taking the waters' had fallen out of favour. In 1822 he produced this treatise extolling the healing properties of Bath's waters, supported by his own case notes and the writings of other physicians. He claimed that manifold afflictions, ranging from gout to indigestion, could be eased by drinking or bathing in these mineral-rich waters. In addition to offering careful instructions for treating each ailment, Spry's book includes a chapter on Bath's history, detailed descriptions and a sketch of the Roman baths, and a summary of the authors who had previously described the baths, from Solinus in the third century to Spry's contemporaries. Opening the work with a supplicating dedication to one of Bath's wealthy patrons, Charles Herbert Pierrepont, second Earl Manvers, Spry also used the book to appeal for the much-needed restoration of the Roman baths.

Cambridge University Press has long been a pioneer in the reissuing of out-of-print titles from its own backlist, producing digital reprints of books that are still sought after by scholars and students but could not be reprinted economically using traditional technology. The Cambridge Library Collection extends this activity to a wider range of books which are still of importance to researchers and professionals, either for the source material they contain, or as landmarks in the history of their academic discipline.

Drawing from the world-renowned collections in the Cambridge University Library and other partner libraries, and guided by the advice of experts in each subject area, Cambridge University Press is using state-of-the-art scanning machines in its own Printing House to capture the content of each book selected for inclusion. The files are processed to give a consistently clear, crisp image, and the books finished to the high quality standard for which the Press is recognised around the world. The latest print-on-demand technology ensures that the books will remain available indefinitely, and that orders for single or multiple copies can quickly be supplied.

The Cambridge Library Collection brings back to life books of enduring scholarly value (including out-of-copyright works originally issued by other publishers) across a wide range of disciplines in the humanities and social sciences and in science and technology.

Practical Treatise on the Bath Waters, Tending to Illustrate their Beneficial Effects in Chronic Diseases

Containing, Likewise, a Brief Account of the City of Bath, and of the Hot Springs

Joseph Hume Spry

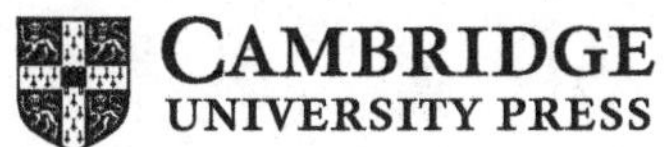

CAMBRIDGE
UNIVERSITY PRESS

University Printing House, Cambridge, CB2 8BS, United Kingdom

Published in the United States of America by Cambridge University Press, New York

Cambridge University Press is part of the University of Cambridge.
It furthers the University's mission by disseminating knowledge in the pursuit of education, learning and research at the highest international levels of excellence.

www.cambridge.org
Information on this title: www.cambridge.org/9781108066372

This edition first published 1822
This digitally printed version 2014

ISBN 978-1-108-06637-2 Paperback

PRACTICAL TREATISE

ON THE

BATH WATERS,

TENDING TO ILLUSTRATE THEIR BENEFICIAL EFFECTS IN

Chronic Diseases,

PARTICULARLY IN

GOUT, RHEUMATISM, PARALYSIS, LEAD COLIC, INDIGESTION, BILIARY AFFECTIONS,

AND

UTERINE AND CUTANEOUS DISEASES;

Confirmed by Cases.

CONTAINING, LIKEWISE,

A BRIEF ACCOUNT OF THE CITY OF BATH, AND OF THE HOT SPRINGS.

By JOSEPH HUME SPRY, Surgeon, &c.

"O BONE DEUS, QUAM PROVIDA NATURA MISERIS
"MORTALIBUS SUCCURRIT"

LONDON:

LONGMAN, HURST, REES, ORME, AND BROWN,
PATERNOSTER-ROW.

1822.

BATH:

PRINTED BY RICHARD CRUTTWELL, ST. JAMES'S-STREET.

TO THE RIGHT HONOURABLE

CHARLES HERBERT, EARL MANVERS,

VISCOUNT NEWARK, BARON PIERREPONT,

&c. &c. &c.

MY LORD,

I TRUST you will excuse the liberty I have taken in claiming the patronage of your Lordship's name in support of a humble attempt to vindicate the medicinal character of the Bath Waters, and to restore them to that celebrity, which for ages they enjoyed.

The lively interest your Lordship takes in the welfare of the City of Bath, cannot be more strongly evinced, than in your determination, on all occasions, to sacrifice your private interest at the shrine of public benefit

The restoration of our noble Gothic Cathedral to its primitive beauty, divested of those appendages which now disgrace its appearance, will for ever stamp your Lordship's disinterested conduct.

Had your Lordship been present at the discovery of the magnificent Roman Ruins, on your Lordship's property, in the year 1756, we should not at this time have had occasion to lament that want of taste which could consign to oblivion the finest specimen of Roman grandeur extant in this nation.

It does not, however, appear, my Lord, that this beautiful relic was at all mutilated on its discovery, but that it exists at this moment in almost the same state of preservation in which it was left in the days of the Saxons. Your Lordship will observe, that I have hazarded a conjecture, that the grand spring which supplied these noble baths still exists in the centre of the large bath; and the more I consider the subject, the more convinced am I of the truth of the supposition, and that the present Kingston spring is merely a leakage from the main body of water. The inefficiency of the present springs for the supply of baths of such magnificent dimensions, the distance of the King's Bath from the great Roman Bath; the concurring testimony of all writers, that there formerly existed a spring under the Priory; and lastly, that the Romans never would have erected their baths at a distance from the springs;—all these circumstances combined are, in my mind, "proofs as strong "as holy writ."

If your Lordship, on a consideration of these conjectures, should be of the same opinion, the public may look with confidence to your Lordship, that what is possible to be done for the restoration of these remnants of antiquity will not be overlooked.

That under your Lordship's auspices the Lower Town of Bath may be restored to its pristine splendour, and that your Lordship, in the enjoyment of health, may long continue the Patron of the Arts, and the Benefactor of this ancient City, is the fervent prayer of

Your Lordship's

Most devoted humble Servant,

J. H. SPRY.

Gay-Street, Bath,
Dec. 1, 1822.

Explanation of the Plan and Section of the ***ROMAN BATH,*** *laid open in the City of Bath in the Year* 1756, *with the Discoveries between the Years* 1799 *and* 1803.

A. B. C. D.	A Bath, 41 feet long, and 34 feet wide.
E. E.	Two semicircular Baths.
F. F.	Two Vapour Baths, whose floors were supported by pillars of brick composition, 1¾ inch thick, and 9 inches square, as at *c. c. c.* consolidated with strong mortar, about 14 inches asunder; these sustain a floor of strong hard tiles about 2 feet square, as at *d. d. d.* on which were layers of very firm cement. These rooms were set round with square brick tubes from 16 to 20 inches in length, as at *e. e. e. e.*
G. G	Furnaces by which the Vapour Baths were heated.
H. H. H. H.	Tepid Baths, with tesselated Pavements.
J. J. J. J. J. J.	were Dressing-Rooms, or Antichambers.
K. K. K. K....	Part of a greater Bath, 90 feet long and 68 wide.
L.	Part of a leaden Cistern, containing water nearly of the same heat with the King's Bath.
M.	A Channel which conveyed the Hot Water into the Eastern square Bath.——*b. b.* Channels for conveying water.
N.	The Western Bath, corresponding with the opposite side.
O.	Supposed to be about the situation of the King's Bath.
P. P. P. P. P.	The Western Side of the Baths discovered between the years 1799 and 1803.
1. 2. 3. 4, &c.	Bases of Pilasters which supported roofs.
a. a. a. a. ...	Steps leading down to the Semicircular Baths.
f. f.	Drains to convey the Water to the River.

The walls of these magnificent Ruins, when discovered in 1756, were six or seven feet high, built of stone and mortar, and were lined with coats of red Roman cement, then very firm. The parts lately exposed were also about the same height, and coated or plastered in the same manner.

For further particulars the reader is referred to pages 16—149.

ERRATA.

Page 19, *line* 23, for *Saxon Monarch*, read *Saxon General.*
68, *in the note*, for *trabentes*, read *trahentes*,
128, *line* 22, for *factum*, read *jactum.*
ib. —— 25, for *antiquitas*, read *antiquitus.*
ib. —— 28, for *Valerialus*, read *Valerius.*
191, —— 25, for *giving*, read *given.*
336, —— 23, for *voided*, read *avoided.*
361, —— 12, for *months*, read *weeks.*
373, —— 8, for *four of the children*, read *six of the children.*
390, —— 21, for *has*, read *have.*

INTRODUCTION.

It often happens that efficient remedies within our reach are little estimated, whilst insignificant ones, which are attended with trouble and difficulty in procuring, are very highly valued. Thus it is with the Bath Waters; their virtues, heat, and properties, have been so long the subject of our conjectures, and, as it were, interwoven with our ideas, that they have entirely lost their novelty, and we cease to regard them either as one of the most wonderful phenomena in nature, or as a remedy possessing the power of alleviating some of the most distressing maladies to which mankind are subject. So much for the revolutions of opinion; and though this is generally considered a wise age, yet it appears to be very much the fashion of the times to neglect the good we possess in pursuit of a phantom, and in grasping at the shadow, lose the substance.

The reputation of the Bath Waters has stood on such high ground for a series of ages that it must be painful to the liberal mind to observe the endeavours which are made to lessen their value in the eyes of the public. To rescue them from unmerited obloquy, and to restore them to that celebrity they have so justly acquired, is the object in obtruding these pages on the public.

The benefit derived from the use of the Bath Waters is not a matter of speculative opinion, but one of practical experience; yet the dogmatical assertions of the sceptics of the day pervert the judgment, and make the "worse appear the better "reason."

Look at our venerable Abbey, and recollect an historical fact connected with it, which ought to be blazoned in letters of gold. This noble Gothic pile for upwards of a century after the dissolution of the monasteries by Henry VIII. presented only bare walls, without windows, pavement, or roof—weeds and grass springing up in the centre of it. The immense expense attending its completion was too great for any private individual; and it was at length finished by the aid of the Nobility and Gentry who came to Bath for the benefit of the Waters.

What a noble testimonial was here! or what more appropriate method could be thought of, than in restoring the House of God in gratitude for benefits received? Hardly an individual part of the church but is a memento of some pious patient's contribution towards its restoration. The benevolent Bellot glazed the great window towards the east, and otherwise largely contributed. The celebrated Lord Burleigh assisted in completing the choir; and one must not forget that a considerable portion of the arched ceiling was beautified at the cost of Hugh Bagley, a famous bone-setter, *parvis componere magna*. The pious Montague, Bishop of Bath and Wells, gave £1000 towards the roof, a great sum in those days; and the Lady Elizabeth Boothe paved the greatest part of the floor of the eastern aisle. In short, the contributors to this magnificent building include many of the first families in the kingdom, who accidentally came here for the benefit of their health. What more convincing proof, if proof were necessary, that the hot springs were not a fallacious remedy? And if (properly administered) they were beneficial at that period, what cause can be adduced to depreciate their virtues at this time?

The principal object in the present Treatise has been to collect such a mass of practical information, as shall prove a Guide to Invalids at a distance, and direct them, in what cases, similar to their own, the Bath Waters have been found beneficial.

To make this plan as intelligible as possible, a chapter has been appropriated to each particular subject; and I trust it will be no disparagement to the undertaking, that each chapter has been headed by a short account of the disease itself, preparatory to the commencement of its chronic stage, (in which stage only the Waters are recommended,) thereby giving the patient an opportunity of ascertaining with correctness the nature of his disease, and its proper adaptation to the use of the Bath Waters.

By the above observation it is not intended to supersede the necessity of consulting the Medical Friend at a distance on the propriety of a trial of these Waters; but it is certainly meant to give the patient an opportunity of judging by comparison, and being convinced through the medium of his own senses.

The reading of a case of gout and rheumatism similar to his own, which has reaped benefit by the aid of the Bath Waters, to the poor hypochondriac at a distance, raises a gleam of hope, which suspends the progress of disease, lightens the fatigue of a wearisome journey, and ultimately promotes that recovery, for which his best energies have been exerted.

It is in instances of this kind that a practical work on the Bath Waters, illustrated by cases, may prove of general utility. Notwithstanding Drs. Guidot, Oliver, and Charlton published similar works many years ago, yet their accounts of cases were, at that period, very incorrect; not from any fault in themselves, for they were men of talent and sound practical knowledge, but from the fault of the age; from the want of that nosological arrangement which has tended so much to the improvement of physic at the present day.

It may very naturally be enquired, whether there are not more recent Treatises on the Bath Waters? undoubtedly there are; but still, I conceive, none exactly on the present plan.

The able works of Dr. Falconer and Sir George Gibbes will always be referred to with pleasure and information; it is, however, many years since the former work was published, and the latter treats of diseases in general too slightly to be of any material assistance to the invalid.

It has not been thought necessary to give any fresh analysis of the Waters. The discordant opinions on this subject will be alluded to, when treating on the various authors who have written upon them.

In addition to many valuable cases of my own which have occurred in twenty years practice, I have extracted some of the most prominent from the works of Drs. Pierce, Oliver, and Charlton; from the two latter the extracts are truly valuable, as the cases are entirely furnished from the public records of that excellent Charity, the Bath Hospital. Some few cases have likewise been obtained from other sources; but principally with a view of illustrating some particular point. On the whole, I have preferred public to private cases, of whatever description.

In relating the cases, for the purpose of elucidating the nature of the Waters, and the various diseases benefited by their application, it has been my aim to give "the whole truth, and nothing but "the truth;" to state my observations drawn from practice, and leave the unbiassed reader to form his own judgment. There can be no doubt, that, in the recital of cases, the most minute symptoms should be pointed out; and it is to be regretted, that in private practice, as well as in public hospitals, we have not always the means of arriving at the truth in these particulars.

The Bath Waters being only serviceable in chronic cases, and chiefly recommended in diseases of long standing, many of the particulars which originally gave rise to the attack are often lost sight of; and not unfrequently the original disease has been superseded by others of a totally different nature. Our only course under these circumstances is, to state as accurately as possible every symptom within our knowledge, and faithfully to describe the mode of treatment.

In the short account of the History of Bath it has been thought necessary to give, many circumstances and events of lesser interest have been omitted. Further light will, however, be thrown on the Medical History of Bath during the 16th and 17th centuries, when tracing the origin of the Hot Springs, and treating of the Authors who have written on the Bath Waters.

We cannot help noticing in this place an assertion which has lately been made by an anonymous author, in the Journal of Science and the Arts, No. xxv. p. 30, attributing the neglect of the Bath Waters to the influence of an individual opinion,* "altogether unfavourable" to their exhibition. Is it possible to suppose, that the opinion of an individual should have been so blindly followed, as to influence the whole of the medical tribe at Bath in decrying a remedy, which is the foundation of its prosperity, nay, almost of its existence? Or, that the *ipse dixit* of any theorist, let his merit and abilities be ever so highly estimated, should, in the face of well-attested facts, induce his brethren of the profession to shut their eyes against their own experience? Certainly not. Neither is it correct to assert, that from the influence of this opinion, "a "great proportion of persons sent hither to drink "the waters have not been allowed to taste them."

We will not analyse the motives which could have induced the writer to asperse so unjustly the whole of his medical brethren, particularly the highly-respected individual alluded to; who,

*That of the Author of "Elements of Pathology and Thera-"peutics."

had Providence spared his useful life, would honourably and independently have rendered his assistance towards stemming that tide of quackery and delusion, which at present disgraces civilized society.

It has been a main object of the guardians of our Hot Springs to render every thing regarding them as commodious as possible. Accordingly we find the public baths particularly distinguished for their elegance and convenience; the guides and attendants are civil and respectful; the baths and anti-rooms clean and well ventilated; and, should any negligence or impropriety occur, there is suspended in every room a printed list of the Medical Committee, (who superintend the baths,) with their places of abode, by any one of whom, on receiving the grounds of complaint, every satisfaction will be afforded.

The material originally positioned here is too large for reproduction in this reissue. A PDF can be downloaded from the web address given on page iv of this book, by clicking on 'Resources Available'.

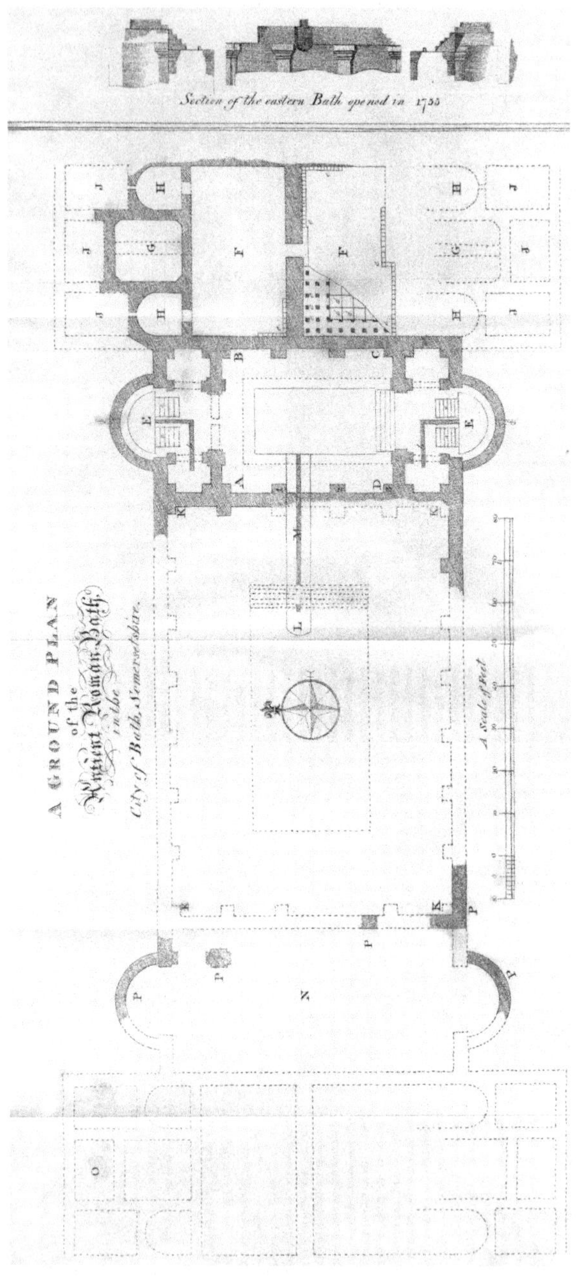

The material originally positioned here is too large for reproduction in this reissue. A PDF can be downloaded from the web address given on page iv of this book, by clicking on 'Resources Available'.

ON THE

ANCIENT CITY OF BATH.

THE aboriginal history of the city of Bath is certainly involved in great obscurity; and it would be an herculean task, and tending to no practical good, to wade through the regions of fable and superstition in pursuit of an object that can never be satisfactorily ascertained. The hot springs were, no doubt, the origin of the city; and the earliest records, both literal and monumental, prove, that Bath as a city existed in a considerable state of civilization at a very early period.

In alluding, however, to this famous city and its hot springs, it might be thought culpable not to refer to the various opinions which history furnishes of its origin.

Geoffry of Monmouth informs us, that the ancient Britons were a colony of Trojans, who settled here under the command of Brutus, grandson of Æneas, about the year 890 before the birth of our Saviour. Rapin gives no credit to the above account, but supposes, with Camden and other historians, that Great Britain was peopled by the Celtæ or Gauls, descended from Gomer, son of Japhet.

Hudibras, the seventh in descent from Brutus, was the father of Bladud, the founder of the city. According to fabulous accounts, he discovered the hot springs by observing a herd of swine wallowing in the smoking morass; and being thus induced to try the waters, was by their use cured of the leprosy, and in gratitude for his recovery, he built the city, dedicated it to Minerva, and erected baths for the benefit of the public. Without alluding to Bladud's pigs, or ascribing to him, with some authors, magical powers, it does appear very probable, that the extraordinary phenomenon of the hot springs, with the beauty of the surrounding scenery, induced him to found the city; and in the earlier stages of society most of the famous cities of the world may have had some such accidental origin.

Notwithstanding the sneers of my Lord Rochester, (whose opinion in matters of faith is of trifling value,) it is not unlikely that such a personage as Bladud did formerly exist, and that he was instrumental at a very early period either in founding the city, or by his influence giving it a consequence it had not previously acquired. Truth and fable are so intimately blended in events of very remote ages, that it is impossible wholly to separate them; still there must be some foundation for circumstances so universally recorded. Is it more improbable that the city of Bath should be founded by a scientific prince, as Bladud was acknowledged to be, than that the city of Rome should for its foundation be indebted to Romulus, or Carthage to Queen Dido? Nobody doubts that history is correct in ascribing the foundation of the two latter cities; yet very few can be credulous enough to believe that Romulus was suckled by a wolf, or that Dido actually built her city within the circumference of a bull's hide.

Whether the history of Bladud be a mere fable and romance, is of very little importance in itself, except as tending to illustrate the great antiquity of the hot springs. Wood, who has entered into these antiquarian researches more than any other author on this particular subject, informs us that Bladud was a very superior prince, who flourished in the time of Pythagoras, and was many years in Greece receiving instruction from that eminent philosopher; that on his return from his travels heb uilt the city of Bath; that it was the summer residence of Apollo, and the metropolitan seat of the British Druids; that he likewise founded a university for them, the remains of which building still exist at a place called Stanton-Drew. Wood, in the ardour of his antiquarian investigations, further contends, that the works at Stanton-Drew form a perfect model of the Pythagorean system of the planetary world. In confirmation of Wood's opinion, Dr. Stukeley, with other antiquarians, contends, that not only the ruins at Stanton-Drew, but likewise Stonehenge and Abury, in Wiltshire, were temples erected by the British Druids. The common people, however, call these ruins the Wedding, from a tradition that as a woman was going to be married, she and all her attendants were at once converted into stones, and that it is an impiety to attempt reckoning their number.

That the city of Bath is of great antiquity may be proved by a variety of concurrent testimony; but whether of the consequence attributed to it by the above author is very doubtful. He observes, "the magnitude of Bath in its ancient state could "not have been less, in respect to the land of its "whole area, than that of Babylon, when Cyrus "took it."

Whatever consequence may be attached to the above legends, all must remain in conjecture and obscurity till the period of the arrival of the Romans, when, there can be no doubt, the city of Bath flourished exceedingly.

The principal part of the city in its ancient state lying round the hot springs, the Britons called it by the name of *Caer Ennaint*, importing the City of Ointment. They likewise called it *Caer yr naint twymin;* that is, the city in the warm vale. They also gave it the names of *Caer Palludur,* and *Caer Badon;* the former implying the City of Pallas' Water, the latter the City of Bath. In like manner, the Romans denominated the city from the heat of the springs, *Aquæ Calidæ, Aquæ Solis, Thermæ,* and *Balnea.* It was also called by the Saxons, *Bathancester, Hatbathan,* and *Ackmanchester;* the latter meaning the City of Sickly Folks.

The first body of Romans stationed in this city was a detachment of the second legion, under the command of Flavius Vespasian, in the reign of the Emperor Claudius, in the year of our Saviour 44. These troops were afterwards joined by others, and for a period of near 400 years never left the city, intermarrying with the Britons, and cultivating the arts of civilization and peace.

During such a length of time, and under the eye of a people who had carried the arts and sciences to the highest state of cultivation, and of whose genius, in every part of the globe where they had once established themselves, numerous traces exist; under such auspices, the city of Bath must have attained to a rank and consequence little estimated in the present day.

Indeed, Tacitus informs us that it was the great policy of Agricola, the Roman general and governor of Britain, to soften the rough manners of its inhabitants, and to instil into their minds a desire to imitate the customs of the Romans. Thus, various parts of Britain were adorned with stately temples, noble porticos, and many fine structures, both public and private, of a very different taste from what had hitherto been seen; and the arts and sciences, little regarded by the Britons before this time, flourished amongst them as much as in any other part of the Roman dominions.

The Roman legions were totally withdrawn from Britain in the year 444, or, according to Bede, in the year 427; and during the whole period of their stay, Bath was considered the most capital city in Roman Britain. In it was founded the important establishment of the college of armourers, in which the military weapons were manufactured for the use of the legions. Had not the departure of the Romans been succeeded by a set worse than barbarians, traces of their grandeur would have visibly existed at this moment in every direction; but the Saxons appear to have delighted in destroying every vestige of the fine arts, and what little escaped their ferocity, was completed by the Danes.

That the city of Bath should have been such a favourite residence of the Romans is not to be wondered at, when we consider the character of that people, accustomed as they were to all the delights of Italy. The luxury of so refined a nation had taught them to regard bathing as one of the absolute necessaries of life; and the immense expense they incurred in the erection of their stately baths and public buildings would be incredible, if not well attested by various historians, and the remains of those magnificent edifices even at this day.

It cannot, therefore, be a matter of surprise that the ample supply of water from our hot springs should have given them an opportunity of indulging in their favourite luxury. Accordingly we continually discover Roman coins, and remains of Roman grandeur, tesselated pavements, sudatories, and baths; for it is more than probable, that every Roman of note had a warm bath in his own dwelling communicating with the hot springs.

We shall here make a little digression in the history of Bath, to give an account of some of the Roman remains which at various times have been discovered in laying the foundations of houses, making excavations, &c. The site of the temple dedicated to Minerva was discovered in digging the foundations of the new buildings at the top of Stall-street, and numerous fragments of this vast temple have been dug up. It was of the Corinthian order, and the portico supported by large fluted columns, crowned with the richest sculptured capitals. Some of the remains of both the columns and the capitals are still to be seen among the collection of Bath Antiquities, near the Hot Bath.

In the year 1727, a most beautiful bronze head of Minerva, or as some think of Apollo, was dug up at the depth of sixteen feet in Stall-street. At the same time were found many Roman coins of the early Emperors. The head is still preserved in the Guildhall. Another bronze head, in the possession of Mr. Thomas Barker, of Sion Hill, (the celebrated painter of the Woodman,) was also found at the discovery of the Roman baths; and is in a very fine state of preservation. It is supposed to be the head of Diana.*

In the year 1755, at the depth of twenty feet beneath the surface of the ground, the remains of some magnificent Roman baths and sudatories were discovered unu.. the old Abbey House. "The "walls of these baths were eight feet in height, "built of wrought stone, lined with a strong cement "of terras; one of them was of a semicircular form, "fifteen feet in diameter, with a stone seat "round it, eighteen inches high, and floored with "very smooth flag stones. The descent into it was "by seven stone steps, and a small channel for "conveying the water ran along the bottom, "turning at a right angle towards the present

* This head was in the possession of the late Mr. Hoare, and appears from the fracture to be evidently broken off; and there can be little doubt but the remainder of the cast still lies buried in the ruins.

" King's Bath. At a small distance from this was " a very large oblong bath, having on three sides a " colonnade, surrounded with small pilasters, which " were probably intended to support a roof. On " one side of this bath were two sudatories, nearly " square, the floors of which were composed of " brick, covered with a strong coat of terras, and " supported by pillars of brick, each brick being " nine inches square, and two inches in thickness. " These pillars were four feet and a half high, and " set about fourteen inches asunder; composing a " hypocaust or vault, for the purpose of retaining " the heat necessary for the rooms above. The " interior walls of three apartments were set round " with tubulated bricks or funnels, above eighteen " inches long, with a small orifice opening inwards, " by which the steam of heat was communicated to " the apartment. The fire-place from which the " heat was conveyed, was composed of a small " conical arch, at a little distance from the outward " wall; and on each side of it, adjoining to the " above-mentioned rooms, were two smaller suda-" datories, of a circular shape, with several small " square baths, and a variety of apartments which " the Romans used preparatory to their entering " either the hot-baths or sudatories; such as the "*frigidarium*, where the bathers undressed them-" selves, which was not heated at all; the *tepida-" rium*, which was moderately heated; and the "*eleothesion*, which was a small room, containing "oils, ointments, and perfumes. These rooms "had a communication with each other, and some "of them were paved with flag-stones, and others "beautifully tesselated with small dies of various "colours. A regular set of well-wrought chan-"nels conveyed the superfluous water from these "baths to the river Avon."* The above account of these splendid baths clearly demonstrates the consequence they formerly held in the estimation of the Romans.

A great variety of images, inscriptions, columns, capitals, &c. have also at various periods been discovered, together with a great number of Roman coins, particularly those of the reigns of Vespasian, A. D. 71; Trajan, A. D. 101; Alexander Severus, A. D. 224; Carausius, A. D. 285; Constantine the Great, A. D. 307; Constantine the Younger, A. D. 316; Constantius, A. D. 357; Valentinian the Second, A. D. 375; &c. All these are described by Camden, and, together with many other particulars relating to Bath, by the Rev. Mr. Warner, in his valuable and able work, "The "History of Bath." The various fragments of masonry, sculpture, Roman brick, &c. are deposited in a small house at the bottom of Bath street, and there exhibited under the title of "Bath An-"tiquities."

* Collinson's Somersetshire.

Though we cannot credit Wood's account of the immense size of the city of Bath in very early periods, yet it appears very probable that the suburbs of the city in almost every direction, in the time of the Romans, were ornamented with country seats and villas. The late discovery of the beautiful tesselated pavement, and sudatories attached, at Wellow, on the property of Wm. Gore Langton, esq; also the tesselated pavement at Bathford and its neighbourhood, mentioned by Camden; sufficiently attest, that, in the two opposite extremes of the city, Roman villas were existing.

To pursue our history from the departure of the Romans. In the year 511, this city was besieged by the Saxons, who had been invited over by King Vortigern to oppose the Picts and Scots, but who eventually turned their arms on the Britons. On this occasion the Saxons being surprised by the warlike Arthur, betook themselves to Badon Hill, where a great battle was fought, and King Arthur made a great slaughter of them, and then kept his Christmas at Bath.

In the year 519, Cerdic, the Saxon monarch, defeated the Britons so decisively, as to oblige King Arthur to conclude a peace, and cede to him a part of his dominions, rather than hazard the loss of the whole. This treaty assigned to the Saxon prince the counties of Hants and Somerset; in consequence of which the city of Bath fell under the dominion of the Saxons, and continued for upwards of 200 years in their possession, till conquered by Offa king of Mercia, in the year 775. The Saxon Chronicle, however, asserts that Bath did not come into the possession of the West Saxons till the year 575, when Ceaulin and Cuthwin overcame the three British kings at Dyrham in Gloucestershire, about seven miles from Bath.

It was in the year 878, when King Alfred was driven to take shelter in a cottage in the *Isle of Athelney*, near *Taunton*, in *Somerset*. His defeat of the Danes stands conspicuous in the records of our history. To Bath he was a munificent benefactor, having encouraged and superintended the magnificence of its buildings, and surrounded the city with a wall for its defence.

" When Danish fury, with wide wasting hand,
" Had spread pale fear and ravage o'er the land,
" This Prince arising bade confusion cease,
" Bade order shine, and blest his isle with peace;
" Taught liberal arts to humanize the mind,
" And heaven-born Science to sweet Freedom join'd."

For a long time after this event the Danish invasions interrupted the tranquillity and improvement of the city; till " at length it assumed new " splendour under the Augustan reign of Edgar, " who in the year 973 was consecrated and crowned " with great solemnity in the church of St. Peter, " in the presence of Oswald archbishop of York, " and several other prelates of England. This "monarch endowed the city with divers valuable "privileges, erecting it into a free borough, "granting it a market and the liberty of coinage, "and exempting it from toll, tribute, and taxes."

After this period the city underwent various revolutions from the incursions of the Danes, each tending to destroy those memorials of grandeur, which had been the pride and ambition of the Romans. This was most effectually accomplished in the year 1013, by Swein king of Denmark; who burnt the city, in his invasion of England, to revenge the massacre of his sister Gunnild. In the reign of Edward the Confessor, Bath in some degree revived; but in the reign of William Rufus, Robert Mowbray, nephew of the Bishop of Constance, who had rebelled against the king, took the city by assault, and burnt it. It was in this reign that the dominion of Bath fell into the hands of the ecclesiastics; John de Villula, the bishop of Wells, purchasing the city of the king for 500 marks,* and tranferring his see from Wells to Bath. It is singular enough that this bishop should have originally been brought up to physic.† He practised as a physician at Bath for many years, acquired a

* In those days the value of twenty thousand sheep.

† "John, a phisitian, born at Tours yn France, and made "Bishop of Welles, did obtaine of Henry the First to sette his "se at Bath; and so had the Abbaye lands given onto him, and "then he made a Monk Prior ther, deviding the old possessions "of the Monastery with hym."—*Leland, vol.* ii. *fol.* 38.

handsome fortune, and afterwards quitted physic for the church; obtaining the preferment of the see of Wells, his natural predilection for the city of his fortunes induced him to become its greatest benefactor. Under this new bishop's patronage and example, Bath was restored to a greater degree of magnificence than before it was destroyed by the rebels. He rebuilt the church of St. Peter, erected a stately palace on the west side of it, and made two new baths for the use of the public, calling one the Abbot's bath, the other the Prior's bath; both of which existed for upwards of 500 years.

Within forty years from the time of these improvements, that is, in the year 1137, the third of King Stephen, the city was again reduced to a mass of ruins, being destroyed by fire, together with the monastery and the church of St. Peter.

After the death of this celebrated bishop, great contentions arose between the Monks of Bath and the Canons of Wells for the priority in the election of a new bishop. These disputes were thus decided by the Pope,—that the see should embrace both places, but that the name of Bath should be preferred, and that the title should be, "The bishoprick "of Bath and Wells."*

The new Bishop Robert, about the year 1140, rebuilt the monastery, palace, and church, and

* This title was dropped by the succeeding Bishops, as they favoured the cities of Bath or Wells; but it was ultimately fixed as an united see.

very much encouraged the improvements of the city. He also erected a small hospital adjoining the lepers' bath, for the use of leprous patients, and dedicated it to St. Lazarus.

The successor to Robert was Reginald Fitz-Joceline, who was a great friend to the city, and built the churches of St. Mary and St. Michael. But the principal circumstance which has immortalized his memory was being the founder of the Hospital of St. John the Baptist, for the succour of such sick poor as came hither for the benefit of the waters; and which he endowed with lands and tenements in the city and vicinity of Bath. The period of the foundation of this hospital was in the year 1180, and to the time of Henry the Eighth the revenue was so insignificant as to be overlooked in the general dissolution of monastic societies. The revenues now are immensely increased; and in 1578, Queen Elizabeth granted the appointment of the Master to the Mayor and Corporation of the city, who are the present patrons.

After this period there is little worth relating for a series of years, excepting the religious cabals and jealousies which existed between Bath and Wells.

In the reign of Edward the First, A. D. 1298, Bath first sent representatives to Parliament; and about thirty-five years afterwards, in the reign of Edward the Third, the Monks of Bath introduced and encouraged the art of weaving woollen cloth, which was brought to great perfection, and became the staple commodity of the city, always excepting the Bath Waters, which had been celebrated by Necham, abbot of Exeter, and at this time were in great repute.

Nothing further occurred of any consequence till the year 1449, when Oliver King, then bishop of Bath, determined upon rebuilding with great magnificence the church of St. Peter. Tradition says he was instigated to it by a dream; however that may be, he laid the foundation of the present noble Gothic cathedral, and devoted considerable sums of money towards its erection.

The good bishop did not, however, live to see the work perfected; and the funds being very insufficient to complete the building on the grand scale he had intended, the Priors finished, it about thirty years after, on a less expensive plan.

This work was barely brought to a conclusion, when the dissolution of the monasteries took place in the reign of Harry the Eighth. This monarch, in the year 1539, having assigned pensions to the Prior and the brethren of the Monastery, granted, or rather sold, their revenues to Humphrey Colles, esq; who sold the same to Matthew Colthurst, whose son, Edmund Colthurst, in the year 1560, gave the Abbey Church, then in a ruinous state, together with the ground on the east, west, and north sides of it, to the Mayor and Citizens of

Bath for their parochial church and church-yard. This sacred edifice had been previously stripped of every article that could possibly be removed and turned into money, such as the lead, glass, iron, bells, &c.; and it continued in this dilapidated state for near a hundred years, when it was at length finished by the subscriptions of some public-spirited individuals. Thus, after a lapse of many centuries, the city of Bath again fell into the hands of the laity.

In the reign of King Edward the Sixth, St. Catharine's Hospital and the Grammar School were founded and endowed.

Nothing particular occurred in the public events at Bath till the period of the civil wars between Charles and his Parliament, excepting the visit of Queen Elizabeth to the city, which took place in the year 1591. Upon this occasion her Majesty granted to the Mayor and Corporation a new charter, investing them with a great variety of franchises, privileges, and immunities.

About this period Mr. Bellot founded and built an hospital for the entertainment of twelve of the most indigent men that should be licensed to come to the city, allowing every man a room in it, during the months of April, May, and September, with four-pence a-day in money; and that the poor persons, thus far provided for, might not be destitute of proper instructions how to use the waters on their coming to Bath, Dame Elizabeth Countess Scudamore, in the year 1652, settled a salary on a physician, to be elected yearly on the 15th of April, by the Mayor and Aldermen of the city, to assist them with his best advice, without any fee or reward.

The city of Bath was, in the early part of the commotions which took place between Charles and the Parliament, taken possession of by the forces of the latter; and in the year 1643, Sir William Waller retreated to Bath, after the memorable engagement, which took place on Lansdown, between the Royal forces, under the Marquis of Hertford, and the Parliamentary forces, under Sir William Waller. This battle, though favourable to the Royalists, was dearly purchased by the loss of a great many distinguished officers.

After the battle of Roundaway Down, in Wiltshire, where Sir William Waller was again defeated, Bath fell into the hands of the Royalists; and in 1644 King Charles made the city his head-quarters. During the King's stay at Bath with his army, he harangued the Somersetshire people, exhorting them to take up arms in his defence, and supply him with money and other necessaries; for Charles always looked for great support from the western counties. However, after the battle of Naseby, the following year, Bath capitulated to General Fairfax, and continued under the Parliamentary dominion till the time of the Restoration. Soon after this period, the wool trade gradually declined, and henceforth Bath cuts very little figure in history; owing its support and consequence solely to the salubrity of its hot springs, and the number of invalids and visitants who resort to it for pleasure and relief from disease.

Whatever consequence the city may have assumed in the times of the Romans, at the period we are now alluding to it held a very insignificant rank. In the map of the city, taken by Dr. Jones in the year 1572, and from the account he himself gives of it, the houses at Bath were very poor and miserable, and the streets narrow and irregular. There was not even a common sewer in the city, when Queen Elizabeth visited it. Instead of the magnificent public and private baths erected by the Romans, there was no convenience at all for drinking the waters, and little or none for bathing. As for pumping, chairmen were obliged to stand on a height, and pour the hot water from a bucket on the part affected. These points will be further alluded to, when treating of the medicinal effects of the waters; we only mention them here, to mark the contrast between the Roman city of Bath and the city of Bath about the year 1600, and for upwards of a century afterwards.

In the year 1738, the first stone of the General Hospital was laid by Sir Wm. Pulteney, afterwards

Earl of Bath, and the whole of the stone used in the building of it was most generously given by Ralph Allen, esq. A full account of this Hospital, intended only for the reception of Bath cases, (strangers,) will be given at the end of this Treatise.

The city of Bath within the last century appears to be reviving from the degradation it had laboured under for many years; and in the erection of those beautiful and magnificent edifices which every where meet the eye, we begin to fancy the days of Agricola are returned, and that Bath, as formerly, may be universally hailed as the first city in "Roman "Britain."

Of Bath, then, in its modern state, we shall now treat, first alluding to its geographical and geological situation. The city of Bath is situated in latitude 51 degrees, 22 minutes, and 32 seconds north; in longitude 2 degrees, 21 minutes, and 30 seconds; and in time 9 minutes and 26 seconds, west from London. It lies in a beautiful and fertile valley, for the most part surrounded by hills, with the river Avon winding through it, pursuing its tortuous course towards the Severn, where it empties itself into the Bristol Channel.*

* "Or ever I cam to the bridge of Bath that is over Avon, I "cam down by a rokky hille, fulle of fair springes of water; and "and on this rokky hille is sette a longe streate, as a suburbe to "the cyte of Bath; and in this streate is a chapelle of S. Mary "Magdalen. Ther is a great gate with a stone arche at the entre "of the bridge. The bridge hath v fair stone arches. Bytwixt "the bridge and the south gate of Bath I markid fair medowes

The city has so much increased of late years, that the surrounding hills are nearly covered with buildings; yet the picturesque views of the country, from whatever part of the town you direct your sight, are the surprise and admiration of all strangers. The soil in the lower part of the city is alluvial, lying on a bed of argillaceous limestone, commonly termed lyas, over a bed of which the river winds. The hills rising to the south and east of the city produce that beautiful freestone, or oolite, which has contributed so essentially to the use and ornament of its buildings. The hills on the north side are alluvial, chiefly gravel and clay, with a poor calcareous breccia. To the west, at a very short distance, the whole of the country is full of the richest coal fields; and by means of both land and water carriage, Bath is supplied with that necessary article at a very moderate expense. Indeed, by means of the canals, great quantities of coal are distributed to the interior of the country.

From the situation of the city, from the nature of the soil, and from the surrounding hills, which shelter the town, and afford a most pleasing and

" on eche hand, but especially on the lift hand, and they ly by " south-west on the town. The cyte of Bath is sette booth yn a " fruteful and pleasant botom, the which is environed on every " side with greate hilles, out of the which cum many springes of " pure water, that be conveyid by dyverse way to serve the cyte; " insomuch, that leade beyng made ther at hand, many houses yn " the towne have pipes of leade to convey water from place to " place."—*Leland's Itinerary*, *vol.* 2.

diversified landscape, the quality of the air may in some measure be judged. It is particularly mild and temperate, snow seldom lying on the ground, and the health and longevity of its inhabitants; which is in greater proportion than most other cities, afford the most convincing proofs of the salubrity of its atmosphere. The uniformity and elegance of the buildings, the cheapness of the articles of life, and the regularity and good government of the police, are among the recommendations which have induced so many families of distinction to make Bath their permanent abode; and we must not omit, what is a principal object in most families, the superior advantages of education, the masters in the various branches not yielding in superiority to their cotemporaries in the Metropolis.

To prove that these advantages have been duly estimated, we need only look to the immense increase of population, and observe the number of new houses and streets that are constantly starting up, as if by magic, notwithstanding the rage for emigration. And whilst every other city is deploring the return of peace, which has scattered its inhabitants, and diminished its resources, Bath has to boast of an increase of wealth and consequence, which must continue to be the case as long as our magistracy pursue their present system of giving it those advantages, of which no other city can boast. —Thus having given a slight sketch of the history of Bath, from the earliest period to the present time, it must be acknowledged, that Bath, as a city, was one of the first founded in the kingdom, if we throw aside all the fabulous part, and only adhere to our knowledge of it from the time of the Romans. It will be then seen, that for near 400 years the arts flourished in the highest state of cultivation; that it was the metropolis of this part of Britain; and that for many years after the Romans had withdrawn from England, it still was a city of the highest consideration with many succeeding crowned heads. In common, however, with other cities and other nations, a perpetual state of warfare discouraged the arts, thinned the population, and threw them back into the dark ages of ignorance and superstition. It will also be recollected, that Bath has at various periods been destroyed by fire and sword, which accounts for the insignificance of its buildings about a century ago, and the small remains of Roman edifices hitherto discovered. Indeed, no vestiges of Roman grandeur would ever have come to light, had they not been hid from the devastating claws of the Saxons and Danes. The revival of this city in all her glory, (adorned with the most beautiful buildings, and not exceeded by ancient Rome herself in her internal regulations,) is reserved for the present day; and long may Bath flourish, the admiration of foreigners, and the pride of Britain.

THE HOT SPRINGS.

The Bath waters arise from three distinct sources or springs, contiguous to each other, which supply the King's Bath, the Hot Bath, and the Cross Bath: they differ slightly in their property, as will be further explained. There is likewise another spring of water, which supplies the Abbey Baths. The fear of injuring the springs, or of diverting their course, has prevented their being traced to any great depth; still they have been probed considerably below the bed of the river, without the appearance of having reached the spring head.

Were it possible to explore the head of the spring in the King's Bath, it would most likely prove the opinion of many scientific men to be well founded, that there is but one grand source from which all the springs emanate, only modified in their course, and that the spring in the King's Bath is the origin of all the others. The large quantity of water discharged from this spring, compared with the others, is almost a confirmation of this opinion; half a ton of water is discharged from it every minute; and only about one-eighth that quantity from the Hot Bath, and one-tenth from the Cross Bath. The heat of the water in the two former is about 116° and in the latter about 112 ; a higher temperature than any waters in this kingdom, the next in degree being the Buxton waters, which are only 82°.

Jones asserts, but upon what foundation we have not been able to understand, than on working a stone quarry at Dunkerton, many years before his time, the labourers were obliged to forbear working, on coming to a very hot spring of water. The above account, if correct, would have been noticed in later times; for it has constantly been a source of wonder, that sinking so many coal pits, quarries, &c. to a considerable depth, no hot springs should have appeared.

The fall from he King's Bath to the river is 17 feet, and the Ancients availed themselves of this supply to turn a mill.

As long as we have any records of the existence of the Bath waters, the heat, quality, and quantity have never varied an iota. Whether the seasons are hot or cold, wet or dry, the heat and supply are always the same, affording the strongest evidence of the extreme depth of their source. A further corroboration is, that the number of buildings erected in their immediate neighbourhood, wells sunk, sewers made, and even a canal on the east side, formerly sunk 20 feet below the beds of the baths, made not the least impression on the springs.

That the hot springs were known and used by the Britons at a very early period, we have endeavoured to prove in the account of the city of Bath; but we have no written evidence until the time of the Romans. It is, however, certain, that Julius Cæsar never penetrated as far as Bath, or he would certainly have noticed the extraordinary phenomenon of the hot springs.

That Bath owes its foundation and celebrity to its baths is an acknowledged fact; and the pains the Romans took in securing the springs, and their erection of conveniences for the accommodation of the public was upon so grand a scale, as to throw into the shade every similar attempt since that period, not even excepting the present elegant and convenient baths.

Indeed, the Romans carried the building and adorning their edifices of this description to such an extravagant pitch, that it is difficult to credit the immense sums they expended; for the Roman Emperors in the erection of their baths considered it a sure mode of ingratiating themselves with the people. It does not, however, appear that the Romans had any idea of the use of hot mineral springs, excepting as an article of luxury, and as an external remedy in various local disorders. They had never administered them as an internal remedy, and it remained for the improvement of more modern times to bring into repute this bountiful supply of nature, at once pleasing to the palate and powerful in its medicinal effects.

We have already noticed the magnificent Roman baths, which were discovered twenty feet below the surface of the ground; these baths must have been destroyed in the time of the Saxons, and the ground considerably raised, as several Saxon coffins, as well as Saxon coins, have been discovered upon the same site, but on made ground several feet above the old baths. The situation of the present baths is of more recent date; and the new private baths, adjoining the King's Bath, which were erected under the superintendence of Mr. Baldwin, reflect infinite credit both on the liberality of the Corporation, and the execution of the architect.

Having thus briefly noticed the hot springs, which will be more particularly discussed when treating of their medicinal properties, our next object will be to give a short account of the various authors who have written on the use of the waters, together with their analyses, and theories respecting their heat; then to give an account of their medicinal virtues, external as well as internal; and lastly, to apply the whole to the Cases which will be brought forward; proving, to every unprejudiced mind, the powerful influence of the Bath Waters in almost every species of chronic disease.

OF THE AUTHORS WHO HAVE WRITTEN ON THE BATH WATERS.

From every authority, Solinus appears to be the first who noticed the hot springs at Bath, which were dedicated to Minerva. The exact period when he lived is not determined; some supposing it was in the reign of Titus Vespasian, while others do not trace his antiquity quite so high. He tells us that the hot springs or baths of Britain were then sumptuously embellished, and accommodated to the uses of mankind. The magnificent Roman baths, discovered, in the year 1755, under the old Abbey House, and described in the preceding chapter, are supposed to be the baths alluded to by Solinus. As long as the Romans remained in Britain, the baths, as constituting their greatest luxury, were no doubt preserved with almost religious veneration; but on their departure every vestige was overturned, and the elegant baths buried in a heap of ruins, and so continued for ages, until their accidental discovery in 1755.

The next writer who recorded the virtues of the Bath waters appears to have been Alexander Nechan, a poet of the 13th century. He celebrated them in a copy of verses, comparing them to Virgil's famed baths, as restoring youth to the aged, and the power of walking to the lame.

In the year 1562, Dr. W. Turner, on his return from Germany, investigated the hot springs, which at that period had fallen into great neglect, in a work on "the nature and properties of the Baths "of England, Germany, and Italy." Dr. Turner was afterwards Dean of Wells. His work is strongly recommendatory of the waters in local diseases, and full of suggestions for the improvement of the baths, for building vapour baths, and for providing distinct bathing-places for infected patients. It does not appear that his advice was attended to; or that he gave any analysis of the waters, although he asserts that they are impregnated with copper and sulphur.

Dr. Jones published his "Bath of Bathes Ayde," about the year 1572. This author was one of the assertors of sulphur, as well as copper and iron, being a component of the Bath waters. He was likewise very urgent to have a public registry, that every case might be noted down, in which benefit was derived from the waters.*

Dr. Jordan wrote a small treatise on the Bath waters in the year 1630; and his friend Dr. Guidot edited a new edition in the year 1668, with further observations by himself. Dr. Jordan affirms the waters to contain bitumen, sulphur, and nitre.

Dr. Venner's treatise came out about the year 1637. He agreed with the philosophy of the times, but condemned the internal use of the waters.

The theory of nitre and sulphur as components of the Bath waters was controverted by Dr. Mayow, in a work published in the year 1670. His words are, "quod ad nitrum et sulphur attinet, quibus "thermas Bathonienses imbutas esse hactenus "creditum est, eorum neutrum aquis thermarum "istarum solutum esse arbitror." In proof of the above assertion, he gives some sound chemical reasons; and he also suggests, that the turning silver yellow is a juggle among the guides, which was afterwards exposed by Dr. Lucas.

In the year 1673 appeared Thermæ Redivivæ, by Henry Chapman. This was a small cheap pamphlet, to recommend the waters; and the only fact recorded, was the extraordinary quantity taken in those days, viz. two, three, or more quarts every morning, and repeated through the day!!

* Dr. Jones gives direction for drinking as much as the stomach will bear, and to walk moderately afterwards.

Dr. Guidot's "Treatise on the Waters" appeared in 1676, and his "De Thermis Britannicis" in the year 1680. As this author was considered the oracle of the day, and is quoted by Camden and others as great authority, when alluding to the hot springs, we shall devote a small space towards the investigation of his work. Indeed it may be satisfactory as well as curious to trace, in a concise way, the various opinions of medical men on the subject of the Bath waters, whilst chemistry was in its cradle.

Guidot, after decrying the labours of all who preceded, particularly Mayow, who refused to yield to his opinion, in an important strain observes, "but "the thing I shall more particularly insist on, at "the present, is, that by God's blessing on my "industrious search, I suppose I have lighted on "the main constituent of the virtues of the bath, "in which chiefly resides what benefit can be ex-"pected from the use of these waters," &c. &c. He contends that the Bath waters contain bitumen, sulphur, nitre, and a fixed alkali. But what he conceived to be bitumen was the scum thrown up on the surface of the water during the months of June, July, and August, and which, when taken off and dried, he asserted, burnt like stone pitch. This scum was afterwards proved to be a vegetable substance, which will be further explained under the analysis of Dr. Lucas.

Guidot evaporated five gallons of Bath water, and obtained nearly one ounce residuum, that is two drachms to a gallon, about the same as some of our later chemists. He gives the proportion of solid contents as follow: grit five parts, salt three parts, marle two parts, common salt more than two, and nitre one part. That the King's and Cross Baths contain more grit, and the Hot Bath more saline particles. He supposes the sulphur to reside with the marle, but only to be detected by the smell. He also observes, from frequent experiments, that tincture of galls will tinge the waters of all the baths when hot from the spring; but if suffered to stand till cold, it does not alter the colour. "That the "sand of the bath consists of freestone grit, marle, "ochre, shells, rubrica, crystal pebbles, and sulphur, "and nothing saline is contained in the same." "That the sand of the bath put on a red-hot iron "plate burns blue, and smells of sulphur. It like-"wise ferments with any acid."

Guidot recommended the Bath waters, both internally and externally, for almost every disease in the catalogue of human miseries. The bitumen was beneficial to one class, the nitre to another, and where it was possible for them to fail, the sulphur came in as the universal panacea; and, what was more delightful, he had good solid reasons for all his theories.

Notwithstanding the above, his observations on the preparation necessary for drinking are very judicious; he advises the bowels to be well cleansed with proper active medicines, not relying on a little manna, magnesia, or such insignificant remedies. On the whole, Guidot was a greater friend to the local application of the Bath waters, than to their internal use; the drinking at that period being rather a new fashion, and all the old cures having been performed by bathing, pumping, and friction. He supposes one great advantage of the waters is their diuretic effect; and we cannot help quoting, as a curious specimen of the age, his theory of water passing through the kidnies.

" The drink or water which descends into the " stomach by the gullett, passes thence, either im- " mediately by the veins that have a more im- " mediate relation with the stomach, caul, &c. or " mediately by the lower orifice of the stomach, " called pylorus, into the guts, whence the most " part passeth by the milky veins to the lumbar " glandules, or kernels of the kidnies, ascribed to " the learned Dr. T. Bartholine, professor at " Copenhagen, as the first inventor, and answering " to the receptacle of chyle in brutes; and partly, " perhaps, by the mesaraicks, passeth to the liver.

" From these glandules, or the receptacle, some " affirm that the potulent matter passeth directly "to the emulgents and kidnies; but since this "opinion seems not to be beyond dispute, as I have "noted elsewhere, I shall add no more as to that "here, only admit, that the greatest share of it "passes from the receptacle or glandules by the "milky veins of the breast into the right ventricle "of the heart, thence through the lungs into the "left, then into the great artery, and so by the "circular motion of the blood is carried to the "emulgent arteries, and discharged into the kid-"nies; where, by reason of their fabrick, aptly "accommodated to the work of straining, the serum "is separated from the blood, and drops down by "the urethra into the bladder, whence through "the urethra, or passage of the ———, it again "visiteth the open air; where I shall now leave "it, as of no further use, till it come into the "urinal, and meet with some juggling and quack-"ing physician."

In 1697, Dr. Pierce published a very sensible work, with a "Catalogue of eminent Cures per-"formed by the Bath Waters." He had practised at Bath upwards of 40 years, and being a man of learning and observation, was eminently qualified for the task. He strongly recommended the waters both internally and externally in most of those diseases for which they are advised at the present period. Dr. Pierce did not pretend to analyze the waters; he was satisfied "by long ex-

"perience of their good and bad effects to discover "their nature and qualities."

Dr. Oliver's Dissertation on the Bath Waters appeared in 1719. He follows the footsteps of Dr. Pierce, and gives a sound practical work, disclaiming all doubtful speculations as of little service in physic, being "contented with judicious observations on their use." Alluding to the various diseases for which they have been found serviceable, he winds up with the following just eulogium. "Upon the whole, Bath is the *Asylum Chronicorum Morborum*, the common sanctuary for "all persons that labour under any chronic distempers; where scurvies, cachexies, and all other "lingering diseases, may be cured, *citò, tutò, et* "*jucundè*, by a composition nature has contrived, "for the benefit of mankind, which exceeds all the "mixtures and compounds man has or can invent."

In 1772, Dr. Baynard published a Treatise on Hot and Cold Baths, wherein he illustrates very forcibly the benefit to be derived from the external use of the Bath waters prior to the use of the cold bath. He also states, that during a period of 36 years, he had seen the most deplorable cases of decayed stomachs, and diseases of the liver, spleen, &c. cured by the drinking of these waters. The Doctor did not analyze them, but conceives "their "cardinal ingredients are *sulphur*, *iron*, and *nitre*, "mixed with a *sal sui generis* in a small quantity."

Dr. Wynter wrote the "Cyclus Metasyncriticus" about the year 1725. His work is principally a comparison between the virtues of the Bath and Bristol waters. He gives no analysis of either, but thinks Bath waters a composition of steel and sulphur.

The theory of Drs. Jordan and Guidot was held to be infallible, until the appearance of Dr. Lucas's work on mineral waters. He boldly denies that they contain either bitumen, sulphur, nitre, or a fixed alkali. This author was at variance with all the medical tribe at that time practising at Bath, and their animosities were carried on with no little acrimony. Without further entering into the controversy between these mighty characters, it appears that Dr. Lucas acquired their ill-will by proving the non-existence of bitumen, nitre, or sulphur in the waters; thus overturning a theory which had been cherished for ages, and to which most of the former writers, as well as the physicians of that day, attributed their medicinal virtues. It appears, likewise, that Dr. Lucas was not a graduate of any British University, which was reflected upon by his cotemporaries. They called in question his diploma and qualifications, and he ridiculed their judgment and abilities.

Though no apology can be offered for the coarseness of the Doctor's language, it must be confessed the public were much indebted to him for promoting a spirit of investigation, and for detecting those fallacies which had for a long time disgraced both the city and the profession.

Dr. Lucas's first object in investigating the waters was to look for the sulphur; this was pointed out to him as the scum which floated on the surface of the waters during three or four of the summer months. Having resided a considerable period at Aix-la-Chapelle, he immediately recognized the same substance he had been accustomed to see floating on the waters at Aix, and which he knew to be a vegetable conferva. This substance, known by the name of Bath sulphur, had been long used by the guides (in proof of the existence of sulphur in the Bath waters) in turning silver to a yellow colour. This cheat was exposed by Dr. Lucas, who proved that all substances in a state of putrefaction would produce the same effect, and that neither the scum nor the Bath waters were the agents in bringing about the change of colour. The Doctor ascertained this substance to be a conferva, described by Ray, under the name of "*Conferva rivulorum capillacea densissime congestis ramulis;*" or the "*Conferva gelatinosa omnium tenerrima et minima, aquarum limo innascens;*" and from the observation of this plant, he conjectured, that "the hot springs at Bath were partly supplied from some of the shallow ponds and slow running springs and "rivulets in the neighbourhood." The invariable temperature and quantity of the waters, at all periods of the year, prove this conjecture to be erroneous. If, however, it could be ascertained, that this conferva rose with the springs, there might be some foundation for such an opinion, and it might induce a belief that the springs were not so deeply seated as we have been led to imagine. But the truth is, that at certain seasons this plant vegetates in the corners and at the bottom of the baths themselves, particularly if the baths are not well cleaned and attended to.

Dr. Lucas's analysis of the waters was as follows: of sulphat of lime $31\frac{1}{2}$ grains, of carbonate of lime $22\frac{1}{2}$ grains, of sulphat of soda 26 grains, of common salt 52 grains, and of oxyd of iron not quite a quarter of a grain, in the wine gallon.

Dr. Lucas lays down some very judicious rules for bathing and drinking, and makes some severe strictures on the want of accommodation, for invalids in general, which happily at the present time are completely removed.

It may be amusing to give the state of the medical profession at Bath from the mouth of Dr. Lucas, (near three-fourths of a century ago,) and compare their numbers with the present time, making allowance for the increase of population.

"There are, as I am informed, near twenty phy-
"sicians, who practise there in the seasons, as they

"are called; above thirty apothecaries, who con-"stantly live there, many of whom make fortunes "without dealing in Bath waters; and chirurgeons "not a few, some of whom, it is said, are occa-"sionally of any or all the other branches. These "may be thought comfortable considerations for the "sick, who need not fear the want of any other "physical aid, in case the waters should fail at Bath, "or their sources be exhausted." Allowing for the difference of population, the medical tribe at that period were about three times as numerous as at the present day; the population then being under 10,000, and at this time amounting nearly to 50,000.

In the year 1751, Dr. Summers, who was one of the first physicians appointed to that excellent establishment the General Hospital, published a short account of the success of warm bathing in paralytic disorders. About that period Dr. Mead had given an opinion that warm bathing was prejudicial in paralytic cases.* To remove so erroneous an opinion, under the sanction of Dr. Mead's celebrated name, was the principal object of Dr. Summers's pamphlet. He very ably and completely refutes the assertion of Dr. Mead, in giving a statement of paralytic cases treated in the Bath Hospital during nine years. This statement will appear under under the head of "Paralysis," and

* "Calidæ sero immersiones omnibus paralyticis nocent."

is highly satisfactory in proving the efficacy of the waters.

The next author in the order of time was Dr. Sutherland, who wrote on the Bath and Bristol waters in 1763. There is nothing new in the observations of Dr. Sutherland, excepting an incomplete analysis he made of the waters, to prove the existence of sulphur in them, in opposition to Dr. Lucas. He was at first a convert to Dr. Lucas's theory, but "subsequent experiments in-"duced him to alter his opinion." He concludes with pronouncing the Bath waters to contain, "1st, the hot elementary fluid; 2d, air; 3d, "spirit; 4th, iron; 5th, salts; 6th, sulphur."

About the year 1770, Dr. Charleton published his tracts on the Bath waters. He selected some excellent cases from the practice of the Bath Hospital, which are valuable as facts in illustrating the beneficial effects of the water. Dr. Charleton obtained 34 grains of residuum in a quart of the King's Bath water; of which 20 parts were soluble in rain water, and 14 subsided. He supposes the ingredients which impregnate these springs are iron, earth, common sea salt, a neutral salt, elementary fire, and a sulphureous matter. To overturn the theory of Dr. Lucas, he defines sulphur to mean "all unctuous bodies in general;" and hence, he says, "if any such can be discovered in these "springs, it has all just right to be called their "sulphureous principle, how much soever it may "may differ from common brimstone." Again he says, "the sulphureous principle of the Bath "waters is an exceeding fine aromatic balsam, "entirely dissimilar from common brimstone." We do not exactly comprehend this perversion of terms, neither, perhaps, is it necessary; if the Doctor understood it, we are satisfied. Dr. Lucas, however, has not been so complaisant; in vol. iii. page 289, he has exposed this subterfuge of Dr. Charleton's in no very measured strain.

Dr. Falconer published his "Essay on the Bath "Waters," in five parts, in 1772; and in 1790, "The Medicinal Effects of the Waters;" also a pamphlet on rheumatic cases in 1795, and a "Dis-"sertation on Ischias, or Disease of the Hip Joint," in 1805. Dr. Falconer has proved himself a very able champion of the Bath waters, and strongly recommended them in all gouty, rheumatic, and paralytic affections, (when unaccompanied by fever,) also in a variety of other diseases, which later experience has justified, and which will be alluded to in the various sections.

The analyzable ingredients discovered by Dr. Falconer are given in the following table:

1. Saline bodies. -	Simple. 1. Vitr. acid, *per se*, very dubious. Compound. 2. Common salt, in small quantity.

2. Inflammable bodies.	3. Hepar sulph. cum calce vivâ, in large quantity.
3. Metallic bodies. -	4. Iron, one thirty-seventh and a half of a grain in a pint of the water.—*Lucas.*
	5. Lead. *Q.* If this is not an accidental impregnation.
4. Earthy bodies. -	6. Selenites, in large quantity.
5. Aerial bodies. - -	7. Common air, probably both in solution or mixture and diffusion.
	8. Mephitic air, in large quantity.

By the above analysis it will be perceived, that Dr. F. acknowledges the existence of sulphur in a peculiar form, under the denomination of *Hepar sulphuris cum calce vivâ.* Later experiments have not, however, confirmed this impregnation.

In the Doctor's examination of the sand thrown up by the springs, he ascertained its effervescence with all the mineral and vegetable acids; also, that when sprinkled on a red hot iron, it gave out a blue flame, and emitted a highly acid vapour, in smell like that discharged from burning sulphur. Indeed, it was this fact so well known to Guidot, and the earlier writers on the Bath waters, which induced them to believe sulphur to be a component part of the water itself. When heated with charcoal it was attracted by the magnet. The specific gravity of the King's and Hot Baths is 1,0020, and of the Cross Bath 1,0018.

Dr. Falconer candidly acknowledges we must not judge of the properties of the waters from the small proportion of active ingredients. Speaking of the difficulty of investigating their qualities, he observes, "the greatest part of the impregnations "of mineral waters are of a compound nature, and "form such combinations as we have no opportu-"nity of seeing, and of consequence judging of "their effects in any other circumstances, than as "contained in mineral waters. With respect to "these, our means of discovering, and our capa-"city of judging of, their impregnations, though "much improved of late, are still very confined. "Even when we are satisfied of the existence of a "substance there, we are not always able to account "satisfactorily for its presence, or by what means "of union with the water it comes to make part of "the impregnation. We cannot always distinguish, "likewise, what proportion of each ingredient is "contained in the compound, or what proportion "each of these may bear to any given quantity of "the water. Granting, however, that all these were "accurately laid down, we may reasonably believe, "from the nature of several of the substances that "form these impregnations, the great difficulty of "collecting these together, and the still greater of "combining them properly by any artificial means "hitherto discovered." His pathological remarks, founded on practice and acute observation, will, in the eyes of all sensible persons, not only do honour to the learned Doctor, but raise the reputation of a remedy, which only wants an unprejudiced trial to be duly valued.

Dr. Wilson published his "Conjectural Ideas on "the Nature and Qualities of the Bath Waters" in 1788, in three letters, inscribed to his friend Dr. Harington. He did not himself analyze the waters, but gives a statement of their contents from prior authorities. He thinks that great part of their active properties may be ascribed to an inflammable gas, which he terms "hepatic air, the "progeny of sulphur."* Dr. Wilson subscribes to the efficacy of the Bath waters in all chronic cases, and seems inclined to think, if cooled down to the temperature of the Bristol waters, they would be equally, if not more, efficacious in the cure of pulmonary and hectic disorders. Experience, however, does not justify this opinion. In stating the quantity of solid ingredients separable from the Bath Waters, about 2 or 2½ drachms in a gallon,

* Vide page 33.

Dr. Wilson makes the following ingenious calculation. "That is, not 20 grains in a pint "of water, a very small proportion indeed, when "we consider that more than one half of that "is absorbent earth. Few springs accounted medical yield a smaller proportion of analyzable "ingredients. Some examiners of these waters "have computed the analyzable ingredients contained in them not to amount to one three-"hundredth part of the whole. If they had said to "one five-hundredth part, I believe they would "have been nearer the mark. However small this "proportion may seem, yet it amounts to an immense quantity of solid parts washed from their "subterraneous bed in the course of one year. "For though we should admit the solid contents of "the waters to amount only to an eight hundred "and fiftieth part of the whole, (which is short of "the number of tons which the springs are calculated to discharge in twenty-four hours,) this "would bring the discharge of solid parts to 365 "tons in the course of one year. What a prodigious excavation would this make in the course of "2000 years, if the waste is not by some means "from time to time repaired!" Dr. Wilson has likewise hazarded some curious conjectures respecting the cause of heat in the Bath waters, which will be further alluded to when treating on that subject.

In the year 1800, Dr. Saunders published his work on mineral waters. We do not conceive that passing a month or two at a watering-place can qualify a physician to decide with any degree of accuracy on the active properties of such waters, and their application to the various stages of disease. Towards the completion of a general work on mineral waters, it is decidedly necessary to state their constituent principles, which may be ascertained by any chemist who will take the necessary trouble, at least as far as our present chemical knowledge extends; but their practical virtues can only be known by those who have had opportunities of judging on the spot. It is highly necessary, therefore, that not only references should be given to authors who have analyzed the waters, but also that the same authorities might be allowed to give the benefit of their practical knowledge in directing the opinion of the public. Under these circumstances it cannot be supposed that Dr. Saunders can be very well qualified to treat of their active properties. He attributes much of their internal benefit to their warmth, and, externally applied, to differ in no respect from common water heated to the same temperature. These heterodox opinions will be canvassed, when treating of the medicinal effect of the waters. In stating the discordant theories respecting the constituents of the Bath waters, Dr. Saunders makes the following remarks.

"Perhaps we shall make a pretty near approxi-
"mation to the truth, if we reckon a gallon of the
"King's Bath water to contain for its gaseous con-
"tents about eight cubic inches of carbonic acid,
"and the same quantity of air nearly azotic; for
"the solid about 80 grains, in the whole of which,
"perhaps, one half may be sulphat and muriat of
"soda, 15½ grains of siliceous earth, and the re-
"mainder selenite, carbonate of lime, and a very
"minute portion, scarcely appreciable, of oxyd of
"iron."

The presence of azotic gas in the Bath waters was first ascertained by Dr. Priestley; and the discovery of siliceous earth is due to Sir Geo. Gibbes.

After enumerating the trifling difference of solid residuum in the analysis of the different springs, Dr. Saunders concludes that the King's Bath water is the strongest chalybeate, that it contains the most carbonic acid, and active neutral salts, and the least of the selenite and other earthy residuum. The Hot Bath water is a very little weaker as a chalybeate, as well as in gaseous and saline contents, but yields more earthy residuum. The Cross Bath water is still less gaseous, chalybeate, and saline, but much more earthy. The temperature, also, of its water in the pump is two degrees lower than that of the others. Dr. Saunders likewise observes that the pyritical sand, which is brought up in considerable quantities by the force of the spring, is certainly sulphureous, but that it does not impart any such quality to the water.

The diseases for which the Doctor recommends the waters are those mentioned by other authors, particularly by Dr. Falconer; and he does acknowledge that in many obstinate cases they have proved of most essential service.

Sir George Gibbes published his first treatise on the waters, which may be termed his chemical analysis, in 1800; and in the year afterwards his second treatise appeared, which more particularly treats of their medicinal properties. Sir George states his experiments on the water as follow:

1. The temperature at a medium in the King's Bath 114°, in the Hot Bath a little above that of the King's Bath, and in the Cross Bath about 96°.

2. In the water, carbonic acid gas and azotic gas in very small quantities. The carbonic acid sursaturates the carbonate of lime, which is evolved by boiling. The following aëriform fluids escape from the springs through the water, and appear in bubbles on the surface:

a. Azotic gas .... ,80.
b. Carbonic acid gas ,15.
c. Oxygene gas .. ,05.

3. Iron in a state of extreme division, the quantities, in consequence of its apparent volatility, not to be estimated. According to some writers the King's Bath contains the largest portion.

4. Sulphate of lime or selenite, in the proportion of ,40 of the solid residuum.

5. Supersaturated carbonate of lime ,20.

6. Silex ,15.

7. Alum, or sulphate of alumine ,05.

8. Common salt and sulphate of soda ,20.

The solid part forms about a 660th part of these waters. The sand which is thrown up by these springs is composed of silex, selenite, carbonate of lime, some sulphur, and some particles of iron, which have been found to be attracted by the magnet.

The principal variation in the analysis of Sir George Gibbes and other analyzers is the discovery of silex; but whether our knowledge of this substance as a component part of the waters will at all account for their activity of principle, is a point we shall consider when treating of their medicinal virtues.

It is well known that Dr. Black was the first who detected silex in the waters of the Geyser; and it is only extraordinary that such a discovery had not been conjectured before, when the basin, from the centre of which the spring rises, is absolutely composed of siliceous tufa, constantly increasing from the splashing and overflowing of the boiling torrent. No comparison can with propriety be made between the waters of the Geyser and the hot springs at Bath; although Sir G. Gibbes, in theorizing on the one, applies it to the other. The one evidently arises from subterraneous fires; the whole country is volcanic, the great stream issues from a crater encrusted with sulphur, siliceous earth, &c. How totally different the hot springs at Bath! no volcanic appearances, no encrustation of sulphur, the springs not acted upon by any sudden impulse, but regularly and uniformly rising to the surface in the same quantity and temperature from the earliest period of its discovery.

In Sir George Gibbes's second treatise he points out, in a very scientific way, those diseases which are principally benefited by their use, including some of the most distressing which afflict human nature, as chronic gout, rheumatism, palsy, affection of the liver, dyspepsia, cutaneous disorders, &c. &c.

We shall now refer to the analysis of Dr. Wilkinson, which appeared in 1811, and which principally relates to the springs which supply the Kingston Baths. The Kingston spring having only been discovered within the last century was of course unknown to the authors who had previously treated of the Bath waters. We have already given a particular account of the discovery of the Roman baths on the scite of the old Abbey House, in the year 1755, and only notice the fact here to observe that Dr. Wilkinson asserts the Kingston spring to be the original source which formerly supplied these celebrated baths. The Doctor's conjecture may be correct; but the Kingston supply must have been much more copious than it is found at the present day. Waving, however, any controversy, or pretensions to fanciful hypotheses, we shall sum up by concluding with Guidot, who says, very wisely, "that the best prophecy is but a good guess." In the course of Dr. Wilkinson's investigation he has asserted that the steam engine employed for the removal of the water at Batheaston coal-pits (of dreaming notoriety) had an effect on the hot springs, particularly the Hot Bath; and he "fears "all the hot springs would suffer, should the Bath-"easton works be regularly employed." There is no doubt Dr. W. really credited the above circumstance, or he would not have asserted it in his publication; it may, however, be satisfactory to know, there never was an atom of foundation for such an apprehension. From the Doctor's experiments it appears, that in 400 grains of the gross residuum there exist,

Sulphate of lime - - - - - - - - -	231
Muriate of soda - - - - - - - - -	84
Sulphate of soda - - - - - - - - -	45
Carbonate of lime - - - - - - -	22
Oxy. carbonate of iron - - - - -	6.6
Silex - - - - - - - - - - - - - -	5
Variable quantity of vegetable extract -	2.5
	395.1
Loss -	4.9
	400.0

The air evolved at the spring consists of 94 parts of nitrogen gas, 2 parts of oxygen, and 4 parts of carbonic acid. "The sand, when examined, is "precisely the same as that which is found on "the banks of the Avon, deposited there from "the washing down of hills some miles above "Bath; both of them contain magnetic iron, similar "earthy ingredients, and organic remains. The "proportion of magnetic iron is greater in the river "sand than in the bath sand." Dr. W. supposes that the iron exists in the sand in the state of a sulphuret. The Doctor has not informed us whether he detected sulphur in the sand of the Avon, neither has he specified the quantity of water thrown up in the course of the day by the Kingston spring.

The above analysis was made on the Kingston water, and, with the slightest shade of difference, coincided with the King's and Hot Baths. Dr. Wilkinson has made some most judicious remarks on the inefficiency of our present chemical means in detecting the active properties of the Bath waters. He observes, "the greater number of "mineral waters with which we are at present ac-"quainted, we are capable of imitating; and we "are also enabled to make those artificial arrange-"ments which will produce entirely the same effects "on the constitution as the waters from their "native springs. Thus the Seltzer spa, the Pyr-"mont, the Aix-la-Chapelle, the Harrowgate, and "the Cheltenham, we can form at pleasure; and, "if any difference, superior in a medical point of "view, from their being divested of the inert and "inefficient portions, as the sulphate and carbonate "of lime, &c. With respect to the Bath waters, "all attempts which have been made to produce "artificially a similar arrangement, inducing cor- "responding effects on the constitution, have failed."

We now quote the components of the waters from Mr. Phillips's able analysis:

In a pint.	Grains.
Sulphate of lime - -	9.3
Carbonate of soda - -	3.4
Sulphate of soda - -	1.4
Carbonate of lime - -	.8
Silica - - - - - - - -	.2
Oxide of iron - - -	.01985
Error - - - - - - -	.11985
	15

The heat of the Hot Bath 117°, the King's Bath 114°, and the Cross Bath 109°.

It will be observed, the quantity of silex detected by Mr. Phillips is considerably less than was discovered by Sir G. Gibbes. The gaseous contents which rise in the form of bubbles through the water, and with considerable freedom, he found to consist of 100 parts,—of carbonic acid 5, azote 95; but by careful experiment he ascertained that the water did not contain any azote in solution.

Dr. Scudamore's work on mineral waters appeared in 1820. " Borrowing from a part of Mr. " Phillips's analysis, the complete chemical view of " the water," he gives as follows:

	Cubic Inches.
Carbonic acid - - - - - -	1.2

	Grains.
Muriate of lime - - - - -	1.2
Muriate of magnesia - - -	1.6
Sulphate of lime - - - - -	9.5
Sulphate of soda - - - - -	.9
Silica - - - - - - - - - -	.2
Oxide of iron - - - - - -	.01985
Loss partly by carbonate of soda	.58015
	14

Dr. Scudamore, assisted by Mr. Children, analyzed the waters in London; of course he gives no account of their heat from his own knowledge. He lays great stress on the discovery of the muriate of lime and magnesia, which, excepting the iron, are the most active ingredients hitherto discovered. Although Dr. S. could have no knowledge of the practical good effects of the waters, yet his reasonings on the subject are candid and judicious. We observe Dr. S. has fallen into the common error of supposing the Hot Bath, from its name, the hottest in temperature. This is not the case; the King's Bath is the hottest spring, and ever has been so.

There are still a few authors who have alluded to the waters, yet by far the most valuable are included in this chapter; we shall now endeavour to prove, that, however, they may differ on theoretical points, they all agree in the benefit mankind may derive from a steady perseverance in the use of these salutary springs

GENERAL REMARKS ON THE ANALYSIS OF THE BATH WATERS.

In the preceding chapter I have endeavoured to give the opinions of the various authors who have written on the subject of the Bath waters, as far as regards their analyzable ingredients. It will be observed how essentially most of them differ in their conclusions on this point; yet in one respect they all agree, that the impregnations are very inadequate to account for the known activity of the waters, and that they must contain some latent principle, which the efforts of chemistry have not hitherto elucidated. That they contain no sulphur, except as the basis of sulphuric acid, and that they contain a very minute portion of iron in a highly active state, with a portion of azotic gas, is generally acknowledged; and these are the only ingredients which can possibly be considered to possess any medicinal virtues. Dr. Scudamore has, indeed, discovered some more active ingredients—the muriates of lime and magnesia; which, undoubtedly, may shew the necessity of further investigation, as every fresh analysis produces a different result.

To the other constituents, the selenite, carbonate of lime, muriate and sulphate of soda, and silex, no great consequence can attach; yet there is no saying how far they may assist in the laboratory of nature, together with some undiscovered principle, in bringing to perfection these celebrated waters, whose virtues at present are so lamely accounted for.

One great object of analysis is to ascertain the general principles of the waters we prescribe; not that it is possible, with our present knowledge, to determine the exact proportion of the constituents, or, indeed, that they may not contain others we cannot detect, yet proceeding and acting on that general principle, we are better enabled to prescribe them without fear, and draw our conclusions more consistent with sound philosophy.

It may be remarked with the greatest truth, that the observations resulting from the analysis of the waters have, in many instances, been of the greatest detriment to their use; that the little apparent consequence attached to the small proportion of active ingredients has raised a host of enemies abroad, who, from a superficial knowledge of their contents, deem them impossible to produce either good or harm.

How far the acknowledged contents of the hot springs are to be considered as criteria of their merit may be very justly estimated by every candid enquirer, who will take the trouble to compare the different investigations. It will be there seen, that no two agree in their conclusions; and though aided by all the improvements of modern chemistry, they are obliged to acknowledge some unknown principle as necessary to give activity to the combination, and which lies much beyond their present powers of developement.

Dr. Scudamore very candidly observes, "regarding, therefore, the composition of the water, "we may with confidence allow it a high claim as "a medicine; and it is but just to add, that the "indifferent estimation in which many medical "practitioners have held the character of the "water as an internal agent, has been wholly "founded upon erroneous and deficient information of its chemical composition."

From the improvements which are continually taking place in chemical science, we may indulge a hope that the time is not far distant, when the latent active principles of mineral waters may be more fully demonstrated. The subject before us is a convincing proof that day is not yet arrived.

Thus we have plainly proved the merits of the Bath water cannot be estimated by that of which we are ignorant; and that the fault lies not in the water, but in our want of means for the developement of its virtues. Dr. Falconer is of opinion that its active properties lie in the aërial impregnations; and Dr. Scudamore attaches great consequence to the discovery of muriate of lime and magnesia. The test of experience has certainly pronounced the muriate of lime to be a medicine of no equivocal character. The evolution of azotic gas, Sir G. Gibbes suggests, may add considerably to their medicinal effects, particularly the inhaling this gas whilst using the public bath: and from the known effects on the constitution by inhaling other gaseous bodies, it is likely there may be much truth in the observation. The virtue of silex contained in the water is much more problematical: how far this substance, in combination with others, may give activity to the waters, it is impossible to determine; but in itself nothing can be more inert, and I am much inclined to suspect there is hardly a river or rivulet in England, or elsewhere, which does not contain a portion of silex.* Bergman asserts that silex has been found in the ashes of all vegetables; of course it must have been contained in the water which nourished the plants. He also discovered it in the waters of Upsal; Klaproth, in the waters of Carlsbad; and Santi, in those of Pisa. Many streams

* Aquæ omnes fontium atque fluminum sunt de naturâ locorum et minerarum per quas transeunt, trahentes secum partes terrarum et minerarum.—*Aristot.*

and rivers are mentioned which have the power of petrifying substances, or rather of encrusting them with silex. That this power exists in the Danube was proved by one of the timbers of Trajan's bridge, taken up in the year 1760, being found coated with agate.

Dr. Wilkinson mentions the sand of the river Avon as being similar to the sand at the hot springs. As we know the latter to contain silex, it appears likely the river water may also contain a certain portion; and we are pursuing a course of experiments for the purpose of ascertaining this point.

It is mentioned by Dr. Hillary, in a treatise on the Lyncombe Spa water, published in the year 1742, after describing what he was able to detect in the water, that the residuum, an orange-coloured powder, was put in a crucible and exposed to a great heat, when a vitrified substance, like slag or black glass, was found adhering to the bottom. This I should conceive must be silex combined with an alkali. How far silex is soluble in water, is a question not yet determined. Sir George Gibbes thinks it may be, and he is supported by the great names of Klaproth and Kirwan; on the contrary, Bergman, Dr. Black, also Dr. Wilkinson, appear to think it is only very minutely suspended, and with the latter opinion I certainly coincide.*

* Bergman was decidedly of opinion that the silex he met with in the waters of Upsal was suspended in a state of diffusion

Whatever may be the principle in the Bath water which is not discoverable by analysis, one fact ap-

as minute as if it had been dissolved. Under so great an authority it may not be presumption to suppose that silex may be contained and suspended in water in so minute a state, as hardly to be detected by the highest magnifying powers. Dr. Black, who discovered silex in the Iceland waters, is likewise an advocate for mechanical suspension, but it appears to me that the strongest argument in its favour has not been adduced,—the formation of that curious mineral Fiorite, and which has been principally, if not wholly, discovered at the mouth of the Geyser, and other hot springs, in volcanic countries. This mineral is absolutely formed from the splashings of the Geyser, or the impregnation of tufa with very minute siliceous particles. I have different specimens in my possession from the Geyser; in some the tufa with very little silex, others in a greater state of advancement, and others slaty, botryoidal, &c. and fully impregnated with silex, forming a perfect Fiorite, (silex 94, alum 2, lime 4.) The inference I would draw from the above fact is, the impossibility of crystallization taking place in the formation of Fiorite from the constant disturbance occasioned by the spring; and that nothing but a mechanical deposit can account for its different stages of formation. Another fact in favour of suspension is one which Kirwan uses in favour of solution. "About "the year 1760, the Emperor of Germany, being desirous to know "the length of time necessary to complete a petrifaction, ob- "tained leave from the Sultan to take up and examine one of "the timbers that supports Trajan's bridge over the Danube. It "was found to have been converted into an agate, to the depth "only of half an inch; the inner parts were slightly petrified, "and the central still wood." Kirwan allows that the timber was of the kind least subject to rot, but thinks it proves to a demonstration the solubility of silex. I conceive the silex was merely, though very minutely, suspended; that as the timber became slightly decayed, it acted as a nucleus to the silex, which was constantly depositing itself on the wood as it was passing down the stream. Again, I contend that the silex in a state of solution would not have crystallized on the wood with the constant disturbance of the current; or if that were possible, the crystallization would not have taken place under the water, unless we pears certain, that its virtues must be connected with its heat and its gaseous contents. The observations of every writer on the subject (however at at variance on other points) coincide in this,—that the water suffered to cool loses its volatile principle, and, in a great degree, loses its efficacy. The chalybeate property, as before stated, can only be detected when fresh from the spring, and if suffered once to cool, no artificial heat will restore it.

In concluding our observations on the analysis of the waters, let us not be discouraged at learning the incompetency of our means to detect their virtues. Of one thing we have demonstration—their power of doing good; on that foundation let us boldly advance, and not sacrifice the real good we possess on the altar of theory.

allow a chemical change taking place in the centre of a rapid river, which is very difficult to credit. In short, it is difficult to conceive how water can act upon silex, when the most intense heat will make no impression on it, particularly when we are assured that the Bath waters contain no alkali.

OF THE CAUSE OF HEAT IN THE BATH WATERS.

THE origin of heat in mineral waters is a subject which has from the earliest period engaged the attention of the learned, and various have been the opinions on this interesting phenomenon. Even in those countries where the presence of the most inflammable substances, and the neighbourhood of volcanic mountains, would obviously lead us to look to such sources as the cause of heat, still naturalists have given very opposite opinions on the origin of the hot springs. How much more difficult is the investigation of the only hot springs* in Britain, where no trace of volcanos, and not the slightest appearance of combustion or subterranean

* The Buxton waters being below the temperature of blood heat we denominate tepid, in contra-distinction to the Bath, German, or Iceland hot springs, which being above 96° are considered hot. Most Latin authors make the same distinction, *calidæ sed non ferventes*. Still the various theories on the cause of their heat are equally applicable to all mineral or medicinal waters above the temperature of common spring water.

fire is known to exist. Indeed the difficulty of deciding with correctness on this point must be apparent from the contradictory reports of men of the first science, aided by all the improvements of modern research. The opinions of the present day are merely those which have been advanced by various philosophers centuries ago, each theory as warmly contested, and still arriving at the same uncertain conclusion.

Reserving, however, any observations on these contending points, we shall begin with stating the opinions of our own *Savans*, as being more immediately connected with the springs at Bath. We shall afterwards, in a concise way, review the opinions of those scientific investigators, and wind up with some general observations in reference to our own mineral springs. Not that in the course of our observations it is at all probable the discussion will be set at rest, for the question does not admit of absolute proof or demonstration; still amongst the multiplicity of opinions, we may be allowed, after candidly stating the theories of others, to draw our own conclusions, and suggest which hypothesis appears most consonant with sound philosophy.

Necham, one of the earliest fire worshippers, observes,

Igne suo succensa quibus data balnea fervent,
Ænea super aquas vasa latere putant;
Errorem figmenta solent inducere passim;
Sed quid? Sulphureum novissimus esse locum.

Guidot, in opposition to the opinion of subterraneous fire, thinks the metals and minerals contained in the earth, acted upon by various springs, generate heat by ebullition and fermentation. Dr. Jorden, a friend to the *fermentative* process, supposes an acid spring running upon the alkali of freestone and snail-shells ; he thinks the acid the father, and the alkali of the freestone the mother, of the fermentation. Dr. Lister conjectures the heat to arise *a pyrite et lapide calcareo vegetantibus.* Dr. Pierce thinks it arises from a spring of water passing through mineral substances, and illustrates his opinion by the story of Mons. de Rochas, to which we shall presently allude. Dr. Oliver advocates the same theory, and gives some able reasons against the probability of the heat being caused by actual fire. Dr. Lucas, investigating the sand of the bath, supposes it to be constituted either of "a calcareous or sparry stone, which, with their "brimstone and iron, forms a perfect pyrite, the "cause of the heat and impregnation of these and "all such-like waters." Dr. Charleton says, "I "choose therefore to ascribe that great degree of "heat found in the Bath waters to elementary "fire, as to its most probable cause. This, if it "exist in any bodies at all, does so most eminently in iron and brimstone. It should seem, "then, that these waters by washing off, separating, "and taking up, in their passage through the

"the earth, the particles of these minerals, set at "liberty this imprisoned element, which there-"upon communicates its warmth and activity to "the fluid." Dr. Falconer seems to think it arises from water passing over beds of pyrites.

Sir G. Gibbes states the quantity of water thrown up daily by the hot springs at upwards of 2000 hogsheads. As a matter of curiosity, he states the quantity of heat evolved by them in the course of a year, above the medium heat of other springs, "would render above seven hundred millions of "cubic inches of iron red hot;" that the waters at some great depth in the earth are at a higher temperature, and that in coming to the surface their temperature is lowered to the heat they are found to possess. He thinks "they are analogous "to the Geyser in Iceland, and that at a certain "depth they would be found to have nearly the "same appearances." Sir George further remarks, that "the regularity of temperature observable "in the Bath waters proves clearly that they are "exposed to a very powerful heat in the bowels "of the earth." Powerful indeed! according to the above statement; if actual fire were the cause, we should all have been red hot long ago.

Dr. Wilkinson accounts for their heat on the theory of Burnet, and supposes it to arise from central fire or caloric.

The ancients were very much divided in their conjectures on this subject. Hippocrates observes, *Quemadmodum etiam aqua, quæ æstate hauritur, ubi hausta fuerit statim frigida est, calida autem fit postea, propterea quod terra rara existente, et spiritu in ipsa existente perfrigeratur, ubi autem haustæ tempus accesserit, stabilis fit, et calida conspicitur, calefit enim ab aëre calido existente quemadmodum et aqua quam non hauritur in puteo æstate ob hoc ipsum calida redditur.* The opinion of Democritus was, that the heat was occasioned by water passing over quick lime. *Quod in concavitatibus quæ sunt in ventre terræ, in quibus colliguntur aquæ, in aliquibus sunt montes calcis vivæ, super quas transeuntes aquæ calefiunt,*" *&c. &c.* Aristotle supposed the heat of waters arose from subterraneous fire occasioned by the combustion of sulphur, nitre, bitumen, &c. Indeed, he apprehended salt water and spring water to originate from the same source, and to have been originally hot, and acquired their various properties from the substances through which they percolated. In this respect Aristotle followed the opinions of Empedocles, who maintained the existence of subterranean heat. Pliny and Agricola suppose it to arise from water passing over sulphureous minerals, and Vitruvius from ignited pyrites. Albertus, also Berger and Hoffman, apprehended the heat to arise from pyritical substances. Paracelsus supposed the waters created hot from the beginning by the Almighty fiat—if so, they would never become cool.

Others ascribed their warmth to the heat of the sun. Thus Rentiphilus, *Terra quæ in illo loco est rara, non conjunctarum pretium, vehementis mollificationis, cui est durities; quare ingreditur eam caliditas solis; ergo calefacit aquam in concavitate terræ in cavernis et foveis quæ sunt in ventre, quare illud est causa istius caliditatis.* Mileus, *Dixit autem quod causa, qua est aqua thermarum calida, non est nisi per ventum calefacientem in profunditate terræ, et concavitatibus quæ sunt in ventre ejus, quare convertitur illa caliditas super aquam et calefacit eam, et sic egreditur calida.* Kircher, Blondel, Burnet, and many others suppose the origin of all springs, cold as well as hot, to arise from the great central heat or nucleus of caloric deposited in the centre of the earth. Spallanzani, in accounting for the substances which feed the fires of Stromboli, and indeed all other volcanoes, conjectures it to arise from immense quantities of "sulphure of iron," or pyrites, which are contained in the bowels of the mountain; a supposition rendered the more probable, he observes, by the prodigious subterranean accumulations of this mineral which have been discovered in various parts of the globe.

That the heat of the Bath waters does not arise from actual fire may be proved by the evidence of no flame, no smoke, no disruption of strata, no scoriæ, plenty of coal, but none divested of its bitumen, which would be the case had it ever been ignited, or served as fuel to the *Bath cauldron;* and a constant and uniform discharge of water, and not subject to fits of fever, as described by Sir William Hamilton, when arising from actual fire. In the course of years there must likewise be a great consumption of materials; thus in volcanic countries the hot springs burst out in jets according to the heat of the furnace, and new springs are constantly forming as the ignited particles extend. This is the case in the neighbourhood of the Geyser, where several new springs have arisen, some increasing and nearly as large as the great or roaring Geyser. On the contrary, in other countries where the fuel has been expended, the hot springs have entirely ceased. Thus many in the vicinity of Ætna, whose ravages are seen to this day, have entirely disappeared.

How coal in any neighbourhood can be brought forward as an evidence of subterranean fires, is most surprising. It is one of the most convincing proofs that no such fire did or can exist; for coal would soon ignite and become cinder in the neighbourhood of an ever-burning fire; and if coal, as some authors pretend, is only to be looked upon as some of the fuel which has not yet been consumed, but the continuation of which deeper in the earth is feeding the flame, how comes it we see no smoke? observe no fire? detect no sulphureted hydrogen gas? Are the gas manufactories so inoffensive as not to be perceptible to the senses? The truth is, the absence of flame and smoke renders it morally impossible for the hot springs at Bath to arise from actual fire. The impossibility of fire existing without communication with the atmospheric air is known to every body; and whenever a fire takes place, in a bedroom for instance, the great object is to keep the doors and windows shut, as the common people say, to smother the flame; as they well know, though probably they do not understand the principle, that the moment air is admitted, flame bursts out. Thus it is with the gas works, the inflammable gas not being able to ignite excepting by its admixture with atmospheric air.

It is the opinion of most scientific persons of the present day, and with a great deal of reason, that the eruptions of Ætna, Vesuvius, and other burning mountains, derive their origin from ignited pyrites; indeed, some attribute meteoric and other appearances to the same cause, to which we shall presently allude. However this may be, if it were possible to exclude the air from a combination with the inflammable gas arising from the pyrites; volcanic eruptions would cease, for it is only from the above union that ignition takes place. On a small scale this has occasionally been effected; burning coal-pits have been extinguished by totally excluding the air, and thus smothering the flame; and though, when we apply the reasonings to such immense volcanoes as Ætna, Vesuvius, or Cotopaxi, it may appear ridiculous; still the argument and induction must be the same, notwithstanding the application, from the immense scale, is impossible.

As we consider pyrites as the foundation stone of our theory, with regard to the heat of the waters, it may be worthy our attention to investigate some of those phenomena, such as volcanoes, earthquakes, &c. which are continually called into action by the ignition and decomposition of this dangerous mineral. Though we consider earthquakes as arising from ignited pyrites, and the inflammable gas, in endeavouring to procure a vent, as the immediate cause, yet it has frequently happened that earthquakes have taken place without the appearance of any volcano in the neighbourhood. Thus the great earthquake which swallowed up the town of Port-Royal in Jamaica was not succeeded by any volcano. The probability, however, is, that it spent itself in the sea, which was observed in most violent agitation, bursting its mounds, and deluging all that came in its way. That it originated from pyrites is almost confirmed by the noisome stench which arose from the fissures of the earth, and from the cataracts of offensive water which were spouted up. The various earthquakes which have so frequently destroyed Lima, have also been unattended by volcanoes, although flame and smoke were visible at the time. There can be little doubt from the violent agitation and heaving of the sea, and the inundations of great part of the country which ensued, that they likewise exhausted their fury in the sea.

It appears that neither fire nor smoke were visible at the great earthquake at Lisbon in 1755; and the general opinion was, that it originated from under the Western Ocean. It seems very probable that it was connected with the volcanoes of Ætna and Vesuvius, as both those mountains were in violent commotion at the same period. Indeed, earthquakes were felt in three parts of the globe, and most of the volcanic mountains threw up volumes of smoke and ashes. The hot baths at Töplitz in Bohemia, where the springs had been discovered a thousand years, and never had varied in heat or quantity, suddenly became turbid, overflowed, and discharged a considerable quantity of red ochre; after which the water became clear as before, but with a greater supply, hotter, and more strongly impregnated with its medicinal quality. The water, likewise, at the Bristol Hotwells was affected in the same way, being for a time rendered quite turbid.*

On the contrary, the destruction of the cities of Italy, as described by Pliny, and of Calabria, as related by Kircher, were all connected with the most violent eruptions of Vesuvius and Ætna; and what is very remarkable, at the exact period of some of these catastrophes, similar destruction attended the inhabitants of Iceland. The principal object in bringing forward the above instances is to prove, that wherever there is fire there must be flame and smoke, and if no immediate vent take place, earthquakes are the natural consequence. So well convinced was Sir William Hamilton of this truth, that in one of his letters he observes, "that it was evident the earthquakes already felt "were occasioned by the air and fiery matter con-"fined within the bowels of the mountain not having "sufficient vent;" after some time, perceiving the fissures in the mountain had extended sufficiently to discharge the lava, Sir William apprehended "that all danger from earthquakesat Naples had "subsided, which was his greatest fear."

Dr. Stukely conjectured that earthquakes were electrical shocks; and Dr. Hales also supposes that they arise from the same cause, acting on sul-

* At the same period Loch Lomond in Scotland underwent extreme agitation; and it was then suspected some convulsion of nature had taken place.

phureous vapours exhaled from the earth; these he apprehends to originate from mineral substances, especially pyrites.

Sir William Hamilton, in his account of the destruction of Messina in 1783, is likewise of opinion that the exhalations which issued during the violent commotions of the earth were full of electrical fire; and he conceives great part of the havoc on that occasion to have arisen from the exhalations and vapours. Also, from the account of the eruption in Iceland, in the memorable year 1755, more mischief was done by the electrical fluid, (which destroyed many persons and cattle,) than from the eruptions of the volcano, although immense quantities of ignited stones and ashes, and torrents of water, were scattered in all directions.

Kirwan is of opinion that the interior of a volcanic mountain is not hot; that the inflammable gas from the pyrites is disengaged, but does not ignite until it arrives nearly at the top of the crater, and mixes with the atmospheric air; "the sulphureous and bituminous vapours are thus fired with dreadful explosions and immense volumes of flame; the coal is incinerated, and the liquified matter or lava finally expelled."

In the history of earthquakes it is observed, that they generally commence in very calm weather, with a dark black cloud visible at the same time; and though the air is clear just before the earthquake, yet there are often evident signs of inflammable sulphureous matter in the air. Thus in Jamaica they never have an earthquake, when there is wind to disperse the sulphureous vapours; it likewise accounts for these visitations being more frequent in the neighbourhood of volcanoes, as more abounding with sulphureous matter. That these exhalations arise from pyrites has not only been acknowledged by most modern authors, but is a fact as well known to every workman in the coal-pits as the existence of the coal itself: his only dread is the fire-damp, which is merely the disengagement of hydrogen gas from the decomposition of pyrites. In short, the explosion of the fire-damp or gas in a coal-pit may, on a small scale, be compared to an earthquake and its consequences. In a colliery near Durham, where upwards of 100 poor miners perished, the following description of the explosion of the gas would be equally applicable to an eruption of smoke and ashes from Vesuvius. "The "subterraneous fire broke forth with two heavy "discharges. A slight trembling, as from an "earthquake, was felt for about half-a-mile round "the workings, and the noise of the explosion, "though dull, was heard at three or four miles "distance, and much resembled an unsteady fire "of infantry. Immense quantities of dust and "small coal accompanied these blasts, and rose "high into the air in the form of an inverted "cone. The dust, borne away by a strong "west wind, fell in a continued shower from the "pit to the distance of a mile and a half, and "caused a darkness like that of early twilight." Thus, from whatever cause the vapour may be ignited, the opinion is, it arises from pyrites; and although a concurrence of circumstances may be necessary to call it into action, yet when once ignition takes place, its effects become visible and alarming to a great degree. A little consideration of the above facts will tend to convince us, that though the heat of our hot springs evidently arises from pyritical substances, yet it is not in a state of actual combustion, but probably in that state of slow decomposition, which, as it has continued unaltered so many ages, will most probably so continue to the end of the world.

In proof of the above opinion, Sir G. Gibbes relates an anecdote of the waters of Aix, which appears so similar to the old story of Monsieur de Rochas, that we rather suspect they are separate editions of the same circumstance. Dr. French, from whom the anecdote is copied, mentions that M. de Rochas, an inquisitive virtuoso, determined to find the source of some hot springs he discovered on the Alps; that he employed labourers for that purpose, and persevered for fifteen days without finding much alteration, the water rather increasing in heat. That after digging very deep they lost the hot spring, and perceived the water to be quite cold, though in the same continued stream with the one which was hot. He further states, that the lower they dug, the more insipid was the stream, resembling pure spring water, although, on examination of the hot spring, it was found to be impregnated with salts and sulphur. His inference is natural enough,—that the spring acquired its heat in passing through strata of earth impregnated with mineral substances. If the above fact could be relied upon, it would be very conclusive.

Humboldt, however, relates a circumstance strongly corroborative of the above opinions. He states that near an extinct volcano, in the vicinity of the city of Mexico, there were two cold springs, which watered the estate of Don Andrew Pimental; these springs were suddenly lost in the night of the 29th of September, 1759; but at the distance of 2200 yards to the westward two rivulets burst out, exhibiting themselves as thermal waters, in which the thermometer rose to 126° Fahr.

Another theory, sanctioned by many eminent men, was the supposition of the great central heat; this was to account for all subterraneous fires, hot springs, &c.; whereas it has been clearly proved, as far as proof can go, on the small scale of our penetrations through the crust of the globe, that at a certain depth it preserves a medium temperature.

Dr. Hunter, in the Philosophical Transactions, has given a very able elucidation of this subject. From actual experiments in wells, caverns, and mines, he comes to the following conclusion: "that "there is at present no source of heat in the "earth capable of affecting the temperature of a "country, which is not derived from the sun; and "that the earth, whatever changes of temperature "it may be conjectured to have undergone in for- "mer periods, is now reduced to a mean of the "heat produced by the sun in different seasons, "and in different climates."

In stating the nature of pyritical substances, and their agency in producing earthquakes, volcanoes, &c. we by no means deny the existence of an infinite number of hot springs which arise from actual fire in the neighbourhood of those causes; but it by no means follows as a corollary, that wherever there is heat there must necessarily be fire; and that there is no other way of accounting for the heat of mineral waters, on philosophic principles, except through the agency of actual fire.

Our conclusions are, that although in the Bath waters no sulphur can be detected, yet it is acknowledged by all writers that the sand thrown up with the waters is a perfect pyrite, in which is evident the existence of iron and sulphur; that although selenite can be detected in most common waters, yet the siliceous sand accompanying the Bath water must arise from a much deeper source, as the superficies of our soil in the lower part of the town is raised ground, lying on calcareous strata to a considerable depth, in which, though occasionally we meet with pyrites, yet it is unaccompanied by silex. The hills round the city are principally calcareous; and we do not conceive it possible that the Bath sand, as stated by Dr. Wilkinson, or any sand similar to it, can be brought down by the currents from the hills; for if the currents from the hills had any connexion with the hot springs, there would at once be an end to the uniform regularity of their supply.

That the heat of the waters does not arise from actual fire, we think must be demonstrated by the absence of all inflammable appearances.

That it does not arise from lime or calx viva must be evident from its not being known in nature; for the fire which would calcine the lime-stone would heat the water without a second cause.

That it does not arise from acid springs acting on the alkali of freestone is evident from the non-existence of acid, *per se*, which at least hitherto has never been detected.

That it does not arise from a great central heat, or depository of caloric, has been proved by the evidence of every mine or excavation in Europe, which have always been found to preserve a medium temperature.

The only rational way, then, to account for the uniformity of these springs both in heat and quantity must be, by the slow decomposition of mineral strata ; and although the presence of sulphureted hydrogen gas is considered necessary to establish the evidence of its passing through pyrites, yet this fact will only convince us there may be modifications of minerals in the bowels of the earth, with which at present we are unacquainted, but which, we have no doubt, will at a future day be developed, as the knowledge of chemistry and mineralogy advances.

OBSERVATIONS ON THE USE OF THE BATH WATERS GENERALLY.

Although the population of the city of Bath has increased within the last fifty years from 7 or 8000 to nearly 50,000, and the number of visitants who resort here for health and pleasure have increased in the same ratio, yet it is an extraordinary fact, that the use of the waters, either externally or internally, has been gradually diminishing for many years past.

As we cannot suppose that disease makes less havoc than it did formerly amongst the votaries of pleasure and dissipation, it may not be amiss to investigate the causes which have diminished the reputation of the waters, and to endeavour to ascertain how far any reasons could operate fairly and honestly to bring into disrepute a remedy sanctioned by the wisdom and experience of the earliest and ablest writers.

If it can be clearly ascertained that the Bath waters have ever been beneficial, and that their properties have never varied, surely no just reason can be ascribed why, in similar diseases, they may not still be resorted to with the same advantage. Independent of the able writings and opinions of Drs. Lucas, Charleton, and Oliver, we have the more recent evidence of Dr. Falconer and Sir George Gibbes, whose reasonings on the subject are as conclusive as they are correct. But it is not merely authority we should consult on a subject, where we may " see with our own eyes, and hear " with our own ears;" we have demonstration of their good effects on a large scale in a public Hospital, where the worst stages of disease are almost miraculously cured; and where the waters are suffered to perform their duties without the interference of ignorance, prejudice, or quackery.

No doubt great discredit has been brought on the waters by patients being kept too long labouring under disease before they have been sent to Bath. This, in many instances, has proved more the fault of the physician than the patient. How many medical men of eminence, in distant parts of the country, both by their writings and discourse, contend that warm bathing and warm water at home will prove equally efficacious with the Bath or Buxton waters? At length, from the obstinacy of the complaint, or the importunity of the patient, he is sent to Bath as a last resource; where, disappointed in his hopes of recovery, he goes away dissatisfied, abusing Bath, the springs, and every thing connected with them. This is particularly unfortunate in paralytic and rheumatic cases, and in those gouty affections where chalky deposits take place in the joints. In such cases, an early recourse to the Bath waters would do more good in the commencement than the application for ages afterwards.

Another circumstance which operates to the discredit of the waters is the number of persons who come here for various complaints; who, without any preparation, without medical advice, and probably labouring under diseases totally incompatible with the use of the waters, "drink them ig-"norantly, and leave Bath disappointed in a cure." Dr. Pierce says, "let such look to themselves; we "are not accountable for them; and if they are "not recovered, or (as is the case with many) have "injury by it, 'tis not to be imputed to the baths "or waters, no more than a madman's cutting his "own throat is to be imputed to the knife, or the "cutler that made it."

Dr. Baynard, aware of the discredit brought on the waters by their misapplication, makes the following just remarks: "Indeed, when men will "bathe who are of plethoric habits and sanguine "constitutions, with a cargo of wine and good "cheer in their bellies, without emptying, or any "medical preparation, or that overheat the blood "and other fluids beyond their natural standard of "calefaction, by swimming, or exercising too much "in them, or staying too long on the hot springs, "&c. there, I say, sometimes the consequences "have been ill. But then I hope he must allow that "the fault is not in the bath, but in the irregular "bathing. And what great cures have been and "are daily done by drinking the Bath waters hot "from the pump, *res ipsa loquitur;* for the cures "would speak themselves, were men mute; for the "fame of those streams has not only run all the "kingdom over, but even beyond the sea too."

The fashion of the age, which despises every remedy of a simple nature, is also inimical to the exhibition of the Bath waters. Every cure must be wonderful, must be miraculous; and scepticism and credulity walk hand in hand, to decry a remedy, which has nothing to recommend it but its simplicity; facts and experience are equally overlooked; and by a despicable sophistry we are robbed of the real good we possess.

But the great cause of scepticism, which has operated so much to the detriment of the waters, is the little consequence attached to the small quantity of active ingredients discoverable by analysis. This has been the handle employed by its enemies at a distance, who mislead the credulous world by starting theories in direct opposition to facts. Thus many patients have been prevented from trying them at all, and others from persevering to that extent which could alone insure recovery.

It appears to me, with all due deference to the various chemists who have analysed the Bath waters, that no great practical good has ever resulted from their labours. In many instances they have proved what the waters do not possess; but what they really do possess, or what gives them their active property, acknowledged by the test of experience, is still unknown. We are informed that a gallon of the water contains $\frac{1}{4}$ of a grain of iron, some say much less, a certain quantity of selenite, and a small portion of silex, with a few other innocent ingredients; and as something new is elicited from every fresh examination, a late author has discovered muriate of lime and magnesia; and we shrewdly suspect the next analysis will prove there is nothing of the kind. Of what practical use such information is, we have yet to learn. I do not mean to bring into contempt the laudable researches of men of science in *endeavouring* to ascertain by analysis the contents of the waters; but when I see physicians of acknowledged reputation, like Dr. Saunders, drawing conclusions from false premises, then the injury becomes of consequence; for we may assert, without fear of contradiction, that the present known ingredients will form a very humble imitation of the waters, and this must, after all, be the test of their accuracy.

If able physicians draw these conclusions from the inertness of their components, how stands the case with the world in general? They argue, "that Dr. So-and-so has analyzed the waters, and "Mr. Know-every-thing assures us there is nothing "of an active nature in their composition, and of "course they can neither do benefit or injury; and "the world is so enlightened and so wise now-a-"days, that if any thing good was really in the "waters, it must certainly be detected, for we are "so improved in science, that chemistry and gal-"vanism are to recover all the dead men, and "there must certainly be a new Act of Parlia-"ment to hang them all again."

Still it appears of very little consequence what are the components of the waters; we know by our own experience, and that of ages before our time, that in certain diseases they have a beneficial effect; and the trial of their efficacy is the only true way of becoming acquainted with their virtues.

What do we know of the chemical analysis of rhubarb, jalap, scammony, or aloes? Are these medicines less powerful, because we cannot detect their purgative qualities? Why do physicians prescribe these remedies, and trust implicitly to their effect? Because from experience, and that alone, they have learned that jalap operates on the bowels, and ipecacuanha causes vomiting. So it is with the Bath waters: the experience of ages has proved their efficacy, and we are not the less to doubt the evidence of our own senses, because we are deficient in unravelling the arcana of nature. The difficulty of analyzing mineral waters has been acknowledged by every chemist; and if we credit Kirwan, the components of sea water have not been wholly detected. He asserts, that silver which has remained long in the sea has been found sulphureted and muriated, although sulphur cannot be detected by any test. Mr. Brande has much simplified the process of analysis, and given some admirable directions in the second volume of his "Manual of Chemistry."

Of all the remedies with which a kind Providence has supplied us for the removal of disease, none can be considered more simple or more effectual than mineral waters. That there are many diseases which no human aid can cure is a melancholy truth; and although the idea of many able physicians that every disease has its antidote, if we were able to discover it, may be correct; yet it is denied to our researches for a very wise end. If Providence with a liberal hand had dealt out certain cures for every disease our folly or sensuality incurred, what check would there be to the indulgence of those appetites, which, if not tending to ruin our own constitution, must evidently go to demoralize society. Thus the difficulty of cure in many diseases incurred by luxurious habits may be considered the penalty of our errors, and one mode of prevention; and beautifully illustrates the wisdom of the Almighty.

That the efficacy of the Bath waters may have induced some practitioners to apply and recommend them as a specific for a greater number of diseases than later experience has justified, is most probable. It has been the case with most favourite remedies; time and experience, however, bring every thing to its just level. It is merely a redundance of that enthusiastic principle which should animate every man in the pursuit of knowledge; and this truth cannot be more fully exemplified, than in looking round on the number of ingenious and scientific men, who, in the pursuit of a favourite theory, magnify every trifling occurrence that can be made subservient to their own hypothesis.

All diseases of an inflammatory nature are injured by the use of the Bath waters; and it is only when those symptoms have subsided, and what is termed the chronic stage commences, that the waters can with any advantage be applied. It cannot, therefore, be too strongly impressed on the mind of the patient, that the earlier recourse is had to the waters, after inflammation has subsided, the more speedy and effectual will be the cure.

It is a certain fact, that a much greater number of bad chronic cases recover in our public hospitals than in private practice. The reason is obvious. Patients who are admitted into a public institution are obliged to conform to the rules of the establishment; and the orders of the Faculty, through the medium of the nurses and attendants, are regularly and punctually obeyed. They have not the means of purchasing those luxuries, the indulgence of which may prove injurious to their recovery; and the restraint they continue under, and probably a family depending on their exertions, may stimulate them to assist in every way the means recommended for their benefit. In private practice the case is totally different. A patient who has been endeavouring for years to injure a good constitution, at length, in a great degree, effects his purpose. He applies to his medical adviser, and feels much disappointed if in the course of a few weeks his disease cannot be removed, and a sound constitution insured. Is it to be supposed, disorders which have been years undermining the system can be cured by charm? Then how is the advice of the physician followed? By whim and caprice: no remedy is pursued that can at all interfere with their pleasures or engagements; and every morning visitor *who has an infallible remedy*, is sure to be followed in preference to those who make the treatment of disease their sole study. The moral of the whole is good: the rich man, by his caprice, impatience, and credulity, rarely gets cured, but strives to enjoy his riches. The poor patient, knowing that the existence of himself and family depend on his recovery, follows implicitly the medical directions, attains his object, and enjoys health.

Chronic cases, of all others, not only require the strictest attention to medical directions, but, what is of as much importance, the active co-operation of the patient himself. In cases of gout, rheumatism, and palsy, these observations particularly hold good. What would be the efficacy of all the baths, liniments, or applications in the world, in preventing an anchylosed or stiffened joint, if the patient, by steadily persevering in moving the limb, did not assist to counteract the rigidity which is often the consequence of acute disease. No doubt there is considerable pain in the attempt, but the oftener the attempt is made, the sooner will the pain diminish; yet for want of such resolution, and such timely exertion, how many of the upper classes of society have irreparably lost the use of their limbs.

The internal or external use of these waters is, after all, not to be looked upon as infallible. Their success must depend on a variety of circumstances; the age, state of disease, and strength of the patient must be duly considered, and their indiscriminate use avoided. Many of the diseases for which they are recommended are in themselves incurable, and reflect no discredit on the waters, because they fail to work impossibilities.

It is a charge frequently laid, that, in attending to cases, the favourable terminations are only noted down, without bringing forward those which may have received injury from any favourite remedy. The Bath waters, though they may fail in curing the patient, can never do injury when properly administered. Undoubtedly they are mischievous when pursued contrary to those indications, of which the physician only is the competent judge. It is the indiscriminate use of a medicine which brings it into contempt, and prevents its being employed in those diseases where the greatest benefit might be expected.

The idea of one particular period of the year being devoted to the use of the Bath waters, in preference to another, is ridiculous enough; and to shew the absurdity, it is only necessary to mention, that the period we now consider the most proper was formerly the only time when Bath was empty; the patients being invariably sent from Bath during the winter months for the purpose of returning and commencing operations early in the spring. Under this impression, Mr. Bellot established a hospital for the reception of Bath cases, for paupers, with an allowance for a physician to attend, during the summer months only.

It is equally absurd to suppose that diseases can only be treated properly during the winter season, as it was formerly to consider the waters of use only in the summer. If the attacks of disease always occurred at one period, then could there be no hesitation in our choice; but as they make their ravages at all times, so the Bath waters are at all times beneficial when the disease is adapted to their use. As, however, their benefit is principally experienced in chronic diseases, and cases of long standing, it may not be amiss to express an opinion of the most favourable season for their use, when a choice can be selected.

Those patients who come to Bath with little or nothing the matter with them, and make the waters an excuse for a little recreation, of course will prefer the winter season, combining the pleasures of this gay city with the ostensible plea of attending to their health. Those, on the contrary, who come here labouring under real maladies; who wish to drink the waters regularly, and persevere in the bathing and pumping, with moderate exercise, for the recovery of such disorders as gout, paralysis, &c. to them the season is every thing; and as in the spring and summer months there is more settled fine weather than can possibly be expected during winter, so I am decidedly of opinion those milder seasons are much more favourable for the recovery of all diseases connected with loss of motion in the joints.

In the great variety of diseases for which the Bath waters may be rationally and successfully administered, the various modes of pursuing their course, and how far what or any medicines may be useful to assist their action, can only be determined with precision by the professional adviser. In some diseases the exhibition of remedies, so as not to interfere with the waters, is decidedly necessary; but in most cases it has been our practice, with attention to the bowels, to give the waters an opportunity of working their own cure. The excellence of the physician, the difference between him and the quack, observes Dr. Lucas, appear in no instance more clearly than in making a just distinction on these points. We are, however, in this place, merely pursuing general observations on the Bath waters, without entering into those minutiæ which will be more particularly alluded to under the respective considerations of their internal and external use.

Before concluding this chapter, it may be observed, that the hot springs might also prove serviceable to the brute creation, were the refuse waters of the King's Bath allowed to run into a pond, or other receptacle. Many diseases of animals, particularly the grease in horses' heels, and sprains in the limbs, might be materially benefited. The brute creation have, in some degree, a claim upon our patronage, when we reflect, that to the swine tribe we owe the first knowledge of their medicinal virtues. It appears, however, from ancient records, that a Horse Bath did formerly exist, which was very much recommended for various diseases of animals, particularly the mange in dogs, &c.

ON THE INTERNAL USE OF THE BATH WATERS.

The internal use of the Bath waters is recommended in rheumatic, gouty, and paralytic affections, in all those disorders originating from indigestion or acidity of the stomach, biliary and glandular obstructions, hypochondriac and hysterical affections, and, in short, almost every disease accompanied by great debility, and unattended with inflammation. These various disorders will be more fully discussed under their respective heads.

Amongst those diseases where the water is contra indicated, may be enumerated all affections of the lungs, asthma, disorders of the chest, apoplexies, epilepsies, dropsical affusions, fevers, erysipelas, hemorrhages, maniacal cases, topical inflammations, cancers, plethoric habits, where the vessels appear distended with blood, or, indeed, any disorders having a tendency to lethargic or inflammatory symptoms.

It has been before stated that there were three springs, the King's, the Hot, and the Cross Baths; and though it was conceived they all originated from the same grand source, yet, from some unaccountable cause, there appears a slight difference in their properties, the Hot and Cross Baths being more mild and less stimulant than the King's, or the spring at the Great Pump-Room. This slight variation of their virtues has been of the greatest service, as many invalids have found by experience that they have been able to drink with advantage from one particular spring, when the others have evidently disagreed. These discriminations, however, can only be ascertained by a trial of their effects; and we shall now proceed to lay down those general rules for drinking the waters, which are necessary to ensure their success.

It is usual, indeed decidedly necessary, that the bowels should be well evacuated prior to a commencement of the Bath waters; for if the stomach or bowels should be in any way disordered by improper accumulations, the water will to a certainty disagree.

The usual and best way of taking all medicinal waters is to begin with a small quantity, and gradually increase it as it is found to agree with the stomach. It would be proper to commence with one of the milder springs, that is, the Hot or the Cross Bath, and take the smallest-sized glass, which is one-fourth of a pint, about three quarters of an hour before breakfast; to sit down a few minutes after drinking the water to let it subside on the stomach, and then walk till breakfast. Between breakfast and dinner the same quantity may be repeated, observing the same precautions, and walking moderately afterwards. Should the waters agree, (which may be known by their lying light and easy on the stomach, elevating the spirits, creating an appetite, and not occasioning head-ache,) after two days the second-sized glass, or one-third of a pint, may be taken, and the quantity may be gradually increased, at intervals of two or three days, till the patient takes two large glasses before breakfast, and two in the middle of the day. In this case there should be a space of half an hour between the glasses before breakfast, and not less than one hour between the periods of drinking in the middle of the day. In general a smaller quantity will be sufficient, although the above is a full complement. The exact quantity, however, must be suited to the nature of the disease, and guided by existing circumstances.

If, after a few days trial, the Hot or Cross Bath agree with the patient, he may try the King's pump, and increase in the same ratio; but if it appear to lie heavy on the stomach, occasion lassitude, or in any way affect the head, it would be prudent to take a little active medicine, and return to the milder water.

The taste of the water is by no means unpleasant, leaving a slight chalybeate impression on the tongue. It should be drank as quick as possible on being pumped into the glass, otherwise the aërial impregnation (in which Dr. Falconer thinks its principal virtue resides) is apt to evaporate; and it is likewise in this volatile state in which the chalybeate exists, for iron cannot be detected in the water when suffered to grow cold.

The period usually recommended as a fair trial of the Bath waters is six weeks, which is generally sufficient at one time. Many disorders, however, require them to be resumed after a lapse of two or three weeks; but as this must altogether depend on the nature and violence of the malady, it is impossible to lay down any general rules. It has been found that many patients after continuing the water a month or so have not felt the good effects they experienced at first; in that case a diminished dose, or omitting it a few days, and taking some active medicine, may be necessary. I am, however, of opinion, if the patient be not confined to time, that drinking the waters steadily one month is sufficient; by returning to them again after a few weeks they will prove more efficacious, and this can be often repeated, according to the urgency of the case. Many patients, however, who come here with great inconvenience, leaving their families and their business, can only stay six weeks or two months; in such case they are obliged to make the best use of their time, and I should advise them to intermit the water a few days at the termination of three weeks, and thus pursue it as long as they stay in Bath.

It has been recommended by some practitioners to leave off the water gradually in the same way in which it was commenced; there does not appear to be any great reason for this plan, neither has any inconvenience occurred from leaving it off after drinking a stated period.

Moderate exercise without fatigue should be strictly observed whilst drinking the Bath waters, as it promotes a more general circulation, and encourages those secretions which are looked upon as salutary. Great attention is likewise necessary in keeping the bowels regular, the water frequently disagreeing from want of caution in this respect. Every medicine of a strengthening nature has a tendency to confine the body; so it is with the Bath water, which should be carefully counteracted. In a few rare instances, however, the water has been known to have a contrary effect.

With regard to diet, that must altogether depend on the state of the patient, and the nature of the disease; if the disorder has been occasioned by debility, a more generous diet may be allowed;

but if, on the contrary, too much wine and turtle have laid the foundation of the complaint, an opposite system must be pursued. At any rate, whilst following a course of the water the nourishment should be light and easy of digestion, not fasting too long, or eating too much at one meal, and, above all things, avoiding suppers. Ripe fruits, if agreeing with the stomach, and not occasioning flatulence or acidity, may be taken; in general they keep the body cool, and relax the bowels.

Although it is best to drink the water immediately from the pump, yet there are some cases of excessive debility, where the patient is totally unable to go abroad, or even to leave his room. Under these circumstances the water may be fetched as hot as possible from the spring, and the patient may try it in small quantities, either walking about his room afterwards, if possible, or else being wheeled round it in a chair. I have known very great advantage derived from this plan, and continued till the patient was able to crawl to the pump, or be taken in a chair.

Many authors have laid great stress on the diuretic effect of the water, and have supposed it a criterion of its benefit. I have, however, never considered it as any particular indication, but merely the consequence of the increased quantity of fluid taken into the stomach.

It appears to have been the custom with many of the old practitioners to mix various medicines with the Bath water in the expectation of improving their effect; thus Guidot mixed *sal prunella*, *cremor tartar*, &c. with them; and others have recommended warm tinctures, such as *cardamoms*, and many thought *sweet spirits of nitre* a great improvement in assisting their diuretic quality. The best mode is to prescribe the water in its natural state, and if not answering the expectation of the physician in the relief it affords to the patient, it is the province of the former to ascertain the the cause, omit the water, and recommend proper remedies.

I would not, however, advise the patient hastily to give up the use of the water on a fanciful supposition of its disagreement. At first it frequently occasions a degree of lethargic torpor, with slight giddiness in the head, and after a day or two these symptoms subside, and the water agrees perfectly well. The above slight uneasiness may be occasioned by costiveness, or the want of sufficient exercise; and it must be considered, many patients come to Bath for relief, who, in the bosom of their family and society of their friends, do not feel that lassitude or *ennui* which, on coming to a strange place, is often experienced. These symptoms may, therefore, I am convinced, be often traced to the above cause; and a little amusement for the mind is as necessary to the invalid as medicine for the body.

It was formerly a custom, likewise, to take the water during meals and at bedtime, in short, at all hours of the day. If the water is to have any beneficial effect on the stomach, for the relief of those disorders for which it is prescribed, it is necessary that as few foreign substances should be allowed to disturb its effects as possible. On this account it is advisable to abstain from food about an hour before or after drinking the water.

Great care should be taken to avoid cold, and in the pursuit of exercise, which is decidedly necessary, not to be exposed to damp, or to get wet in the feet, causing a check of perspiration; for if the patient by any imprudence gets cold, an immediate stop is put to the course of the waters.

I have before alluded to amusement of the mind, which should be attended to by the patient as one great means of relieving the body. We should, however, on this point avoid all extremes, and in the pursuit of rational pleasures not overstep that boundary which would disturb the whole animal economy. The mind should be kept perfectly at ease, and every cause of irritation avoided, which can only tend to aggravate disease.

How difficult this doctrine is to be pursued by gouty and other patients, where the irritability of the nerves is considered a symptom of the disorder, we are well aware. But every one must have observed, in the circle of their own acquaintance, how much better some patients will bear pain and suffering than others. This may in part arise from physical constitution ; but much may be done by exerting the energies of our own mind in withstanding those violent sallies of passion and ill-humour, which are too often the concomitants of continued disease, and which ultimately recoil on ourselves.

These observations may appear trifling, but their truth is no less evident ; and that patient will most effectually second the views of his professional adviser, and assist his own recovery, who endeavours to allay the fever of the mind.

Having thus given an account how the water should be used, we have only to guard patients against taking it unadvisedly ; for as the water has the power of being very beneficial when properly administered, so in cases where it is injudiciously pursued it may prove of the greatest injury.

Having laid down the above general observations for the trial of the waters, it may be amusing, as well as instructive, to state the mode of practice recommended by our forefathers, and compare it with the supposed improvements of the present day.

It appears that the Bath waters were formerly only used externally ; and the earliest account of drinking them is in Jones's work, in the year 1572. In it he gives directions for taking as much as the stomach will bear at all hours of the day, for the purpose, as he observes, of "quenching thirst, and "keeping soluble;" which latter effect was increased by the addition of a little common salt. By later writers the drinking was designated a new system, and disapproved by many, particularly by Dr. Venner. Guidot likewise, though he recommends them in some instances, seems to be treading on forbidden ground. He proposes some very difficult "questions, whether the leap year hath any malign "influence on drinking the waters, and whether "they may be safely used in the dog-days!!"

Guidot's objection appeared to arise from the immense quantities of the Bath water which was poured into the stomach by quarts and gallons; and the novelty of drinking was carried to such a height, that the patients supposed their cures were to be performed without the aid of bathing or pumping, and neglected those latter means to save trouble, and gain health *on easier terms.* His lamentations are thus quaintly expressed:

"And whereas the bath in former times, dis- "creetly used, did quicken the circulation, pro- "mote nutrition, cure atrophies, strengthen "weaknesses, confirm relaxations, and relax con-

" tractions of the tendons and all the nervous " tribe; the nutritive juice and relaxed paralytic " fibres are now so diluted, and beyond all mea- " sure softened with a deluge of the waters taken " inwardly, that whatever good it may do persons " in *statu neutro*, neither sick nor well, the good " effects which were wont to be produced by exter- " nal applications of the water to the part affected, " are now frustrate; cures not so numerous, and " if any, performed in much longer time, since " the use of the bath hath become so much in- " feriour to the drinking of the water; and the " diseases formerly cured according to ancient " method safely, quickly, and with ease to the " patient, must now expect the *omnipotent means* " that first attended the propagation of the christ- " ian religion, and not a *cure without a miracle*."

The poor Doctor's complaints were very just; but many moderns think we have fallen into the opposite extreme. Dr. Lucas is of opinion the cures were more numerous when the quantity drank was greater; and Dr. Falconer thinks a larger quantity might be more beneficial.

To shew, however, the little knowledge many of the ancients possessed of the nature and properties of the Bath water, one author particularly recommends the drinkers not to take it too hot from the pump, but suffer it to cool a little, that so the gas may not offend the head.

According, however, to the most accurate accounts, bathing was the principal use that was made of the waters at the beginning of the reign of Queen Elizabeth, at which time they were drunk by a few only; and the invalids were supplied with water "laded out of the full cisterns early in the morning, after the baths were clean, and before the bathers went into them."

Dr. Jordan likewise observes, that he is sorry he cannot recommend the internal use of the waters as they desire, as he cannot be assured that people can have the waters pure from the spring without mixing with the waters of the bath.

The occasion, however, which brought the Bath waters into great repute as an internal remedy was the sanction and recommendation of Sir Alexander Frayser, who, in the year 1663, attended Queen Catherine, consort of Charles II. to Bath as chief physician. Previous to this period the London physicians had usually recommended the waters at Bourbon; but from Sir Alexander's investigation and observations of their good effects, he was convinced every advantage might be derived from their use, which had been attributed to the waters at Bourbon.

By the advice of Sir A. Frayser, proper reservoirs and pumps were laid down to draw the water pure from the spring. Yet at this period there was no pump-room or covered way for drinking the water, but every one repaired to an open pump by the side of the Queen's Bath, which, from its exposed situation, in bad weather made the patients very liable to take cold. This inconvenience was remedied a few years afterwards by the erection of a small pump-room for the accommodation of the drinkers, on the site of the present magnificent building.

Since the above period we trust every convenience has been adopted which can promote the comfort of the invalid; and we are convinced a much more rational method has been substituted for those enormous quantities of the Bath waters, which must have defeated the object for which they were intended.

Having finished our general directions for the internal exhibition of the waters, the next object is to consider their external application; which may be classed under seven distinct heads, viz.

1st, General Bathing.
2d, Pumping.
3d, Vapour Bath.
4th, Shower Bath.
5th, Injection Bath.
6th, Pediluvium.
7th, Hip Bath.

ON THE EXTERNAL APPLICATION OF THE BATH WATERS.

I. General Bathing.

The subject of this chapter is General Bathing in opposition to partial bathing, such as Pumping, the Hip Bath, Pediluvium, &c. The first object will be to point out the diseases in which general bathing is principally recommended; 2dly, the various Baths, and their respective temperature; and 3dly, the most consistent and approved mode of their application.

Warm bathing is highly beneficial in all paralytic, gouty, and chronic rheumatic affections; in all contractions or lameness arising from the above disorders; in sprains or local injuries from whatever cause, if unattended with inflammation; in cutaneous diseases; in biliary and glandular obstructions; and most decidedly in uterine affections,

The particular advantages of bathing in these disorders, in combination with drinking and pumping, (and whatever other means may be deemed necessary to assist the efficacy of the waters,) will be found under their respective sections. All those complaints we have alluded to as objectionable in the drinking of the waters, receive injury likewise from the bathing; and the observation will equally apply to every use of the Bath waters, that inflammatory symptoms are a decided objection.

Previous to our general directions for the use of the Baths, we shall give some account of the Baths themselves, which are divided into the public and the private. We shall also briefly state those other accommodations for the benefit of the public, which, although alluded to in their proper places, are nevertheless attached to the various Baths.

THE KING's BATH

is an oblong square, 66 feet in length, and 41 in breadth; it is environed by a stone parapet, and contains three recesses for the accommodation of bathers. There are likewise four dressing-rooms and four entrances, two for gentlemen and two for ladies. The natural heat of the spring of the King's Bath is about 116°, and it throws up three hogsheads of water in a minute : the depth of the water is four feet seven inches. In the centre of the King's Bath rises a conical cylinder of Bath stone, erected over the spring, through which the water is admitted into the bath; still it is easy to observe that the springs rise in all directions immediately outside this cylinder, though the largest volume of water is ejected from within it. The pipes which supply the Pump-Room are fixed in the cylinder, several feet below the bottom of the bath. An old statue of King Bladud, with a suitable inscription as the founder of the baths, adorns the south side of this bath. This public bath contains, when full, 314 tons and 36 gallons.

Attached to the King's Bath is a pump, for the purpose of directing the hot water by means of a flexible tube to any part of the body *whilst in the bath;* this is called the *wet pump.*

Notwithstanding the natural heat of this spring is 116°, yet the heat generally in the middle of the bath is little more than 100°, excepting over the spring; and at the sides about 98°. This is occasioned by the exposure to the air, and the length of time in filling; and is intentionally so modified, as the natural heat would in most cases be very prejudicial.

THE QUEEN's BATH

is an appendage of the King's, supplied with water from the same spring, and communicating by an arched way. It is a square of 25 feet, and contains two recesses. There are likewise three dressing-rooms and three entrances. The heat of this bath is about 96°. This and the King's Bath are emptied every day at twelve o'clock, and filled again by the next morning; both baths fill in eleven hours and five minutes; there is, however, a method of delaying the springs filling them, for the purpose of being cooler in very warm weather. The hours of bathing in the King's and Queen's Baths are from six in the morning till eleven in the forenoon, Sundays excepted. The Queen's Bath contains, when full, 81 tons 3 hogsheads and 11 gallons.

The Queen's Bath was originally constructed by Mr. Bellot as a temperate bath for the use of the public, and received the overflowings of the King's Bath; but by an opening in the wall it has been united to the latter, and received its present appellation on account of the Queen of James I. bathing in it. Her Majesty, it is related, was frightened by some meteoric appearance in the King's Bath, and could not be prevailed upon to use it again. On this occasion the citizens erected a magnificent tower or cross in the centre of the Queen's Bath, which has, however, been taken down some years.

THE NEW PRIVATE BATHS,

which are supplied by the King's Bath, are four in number, each accommodated with a dressing-room adjoining. The depth of each bath is four feet seven inches, the length nine feet eight inches, and the width, from shoulder to shoulder, six feet. Each bath contains about 13 hogsheads, and may be ordered at any temperature under 113°. There is also a pump passing into each bath, should it be required.

There are likewise two other pumps, one for ladies and the other for gentlemen, called dry pumps, because they are used locally, without the warm bath; also dressing-rooms adjoining. Attached to one of the dressing-rooms is an injecting machine, of most convenient construction, also closets, and every convenience the invalid can possibly require. The Private Baths can be supplied at a very short notice; and the process of filling them may be inspected by the invalid or their attendants, if they wish it.

THE CROSS BATH

is a small open bath at the bottom of Bath-street, of a triangular shape. It contains two recesses and a pump; there are also three dressing-rooms. The temperature is from 94° to 96°. It is used for public bathing at the same hours as the other public baths; it takes fifteen or sixteen hours filling. There are no private baths attached. It contains 53 tons and 47 gallons.

This bath acquired its name from a very curious cross or pillar erected by John Earl of Melfort,

Secretary of State to King James II. in consequence of the prolific powers of the waters proving successful in her Majesty's case. This cross was of marble, of a circular construction, having in its circumference three Corinthian columns, crowned with an hexagonal dome. It was very richly sculptured, with appropriate inscriptions, and is said to have cost upwards of £1500. It was taken down in the year 1783, when the bath was repaired. There is a small but elegant pump-room attached to these springs, forming the termination of Bath-street.

THE HOT BATH,

more commonly known as the Hetling, or the Old Corporation Baths. This spring received its appellation from being considered the highest in temperature; which does not however exceed that of the spring at the King's Bath, whatever it might have done formerly, and the same observation was made by authors 200 years ago.

The public bath supplied by this spring is a small open bath, built originally by Robert the first Bishop of Bath and Wells, for the accommodation of leprous cases, thence denominated the Leper's Bath. The water in the open bath is upwards of 100°. It is principally used by the Hospital and Dispensary patients; though private individuals may have the benefit of it from five till nine in the morning. It is accommodated with a pump, and separate days are appropriated for the bathing of men and women. It contains 54 tons and 27 gallons of water.

THE HETLING PRIVATE BATHS,

supplied by these springs, are four in number, with dressing-rooms adjoining, and pumps in each bath. These baths are rather larger than those at the King's, and contain about sixteen hogsheads of water. They are 4½ feet deep, 12 feet long, and 7 feet 3 inches from shoulder to shoulder. They can be heated to any temperature under 113°.

One very great advantage attending these baths is the convenience of an invalid chair for assisting cripples in bathing. The patient seats himself in the chair, and by the assistance of a crane is let down into the bath, and after a sufficient time drawn up in the same way, without the smallest exertion or fatigue.

There is likewise a dry pump, and a shower bath, with dressing-room adjoining, which may be ordered at any temperature, and contains from one to fourteen gallons. An injecting machine, similar to the one at the King's Bath, and dressing-room, with a closet contiguous, also form part of the conveniences of these long-established baths. A vapour bath has of late years been added to the accommodations, which will be considered when alluding to the medicinal effects of steam.

There is a neat pump-room at the bottom of Hetling-Court, supplied by these springs, at which numbers of patients drink, preparatory to the use of the stronger water at the King's pump.*

Although the public baths are not open for the reception of patients on Sundays, yet in cases of emergency or necessity, signed by any medical gentleman, the private baths can be procured on that day; still it is expected that cases of little moment may interfere as rarely as possible with the hours of divine service.

Thus having given a concise account of the different baths and their properties, we shall proceed to lay down some general rules for their mode of application, always premising that every case of disease must have a discretionary treatment, and that our present observations can only be applied in a general sense.

In those observations we shall make no distinction between public and private baths, but more particularly allude to the former; as we consider the latter only used by those whose delicate state

* Every person bathing in the public bath pays 1s. 6d. each time; in the private bath, vapour bath, or sweating room, 3s. Bathing in the private bath, and afterwards using the sweating-room or vapour bath, 4s.; pumping in the bath, 3d. for every 100 strokes, and at the dry pump 6d. for every hundred; for the shower bath, 1s. 6d.; for the use of the injecting machine, 2s. 6d. Dresses and towels included in the above terms.

and feelings do not allow of their undergoing (what may be conceived) so public an exhibition.

As it is necessary, preparatory to drinking the waters, to prepare the patient by some active opening medicine, so it is equally necessary, prior to bathing, to evacuate the bowels freely ; and if the patient is of a florid complexion and full of blood, with a disposition to inflammatory action, bleeding and moderate diet may also be beneficial.

The time of bathing generally considered most salutary is in the morning early ; the patient may at first remain in ten or fifteen minutes, and the time may be afterwards increased as it appears to agree. Hippocrates particularly advises that we should not bathe immediately after eating, nor eat immediately after bathing. If the state of health will allow, and the weather is fine, walking to the bath, and returning in a chair, will be advisable.

At first the bathing may be pursued twice a week, and afterwards three times ; this must, however, depend on the nature of the disease, and those other means to be pursued in conjunction with it. After bathing the patient should go home, and keep quiet or lie on a sofa for an hour ; but not go to bed and encourage perspiration, as was formerly advised, the object being to strengthen and invigorate the system.

The patient should not confine himself to the house after remaining quiet for an hour or two, but should take exercise, and go about as usual, if the weather be not unfavourable. Care should be taken to avoid cold, and not to stand talking in the streets; as it must be evident that after bathing there is more susceptibility, and great numbers of rheumatic affections may date their origin from exposure to draughts of cold air. In other cases, however, where sweating is desired, the patient may bathe in the evening, and afterwards go to bed to encourage perspiration.

The time of remaining in the bath may be specified, but must in some degree depend on the effect produced on the patient. If the bath produce no unusual symptoms of restlessness or irritation, with dry tongue and feverish head-ache, or if the patient do not appear oppressed with faintness or giddiness in the head, then it may be presumed to agree.

Many of the above symptoms do at first occur in a slight degree, but subside after a few baths. On which account the time of remaining in should be moderate at first, and only increased as it decidedly agrees. Twenty or thirty minutes are considered a sufficient time for many diseases and persons of delicate habits; others, however, can bear a much longer period; and I am of opinion many cases will bear an hour or two in the bath, and derive more advantage than from a shorter time.

In local affections of the limbs and joints this plan is particularly serviceable.

Invalids labouring under chronic rheumatism or paralysis bear a high degree of temperature best; but it is in a moderate bath, about 96°, that patients can stay in for any considerable length of time. Galen thought warm baths of great service to old men and children, but cold baths injurious.

The warm bath discreetly used does not relax the body, diminish the strength, or exhaust the spirits, even in persons previously reduced, and greatly weakened by disease, for after remaining twenty or thirty minutes they come out of the bath refreshed, and their spirits lighter and more cheerful. Dr. Lucas, alluding to their external use, says, " the Bath waters, from the nature of " their contents, are found particularly beneficial " in a relaxed state of the fibres, by bracing and " strengthening the solids."

For a great variety of local diseases, in which the use of the bath is recommended, other means are most frequently added, such as pumping in the bath on the part affected, or the application of the dry pump the intermediate days of bathing. It is also necessary for the patient in these local disorders to use the flesh-brush whilst in the bath, and constantly move about, making every endeavour to restore a limb, remove rigidity, or promote absorption.

Friction in the warm bath stimulates the muscular fibres, and excites a more powerful action; thus it is particularly serviceable in all ædematous swellings, by increasing the action of the absorbent vessels. Delicate women, and those especially who have suffered from weakening complaints or frequent miscarriages, will derive great benefit from the use of the bath; and repeated instances could be adduced where bathing to an advanced stage of pregnancy has prevented those accidents which too often recur about the same period.

We should lay much more stress on these points, but as the disorders for which these remedies are recommended will shortly come under consideration, then will be the time to enforce them with more effect.

As a luxury, the use of the bath is particularly grateful; and the refreshment experienced after violent fatigue, travelling, or sitting up at night, is most invigorating. In the baths abroad it is the custom for people in health to remain in many hours: this is the case at Carlsbad; in one corner you see a nest of politicians reading the news, in another a floating tray, with coffee, &c. When Louis XVIII. was in Bath, a few years since, his attendants went into the bath every morning; and they enjoyed it so much, that the difficulty was in getting them out again.

It is almost impossible to mention any certain time for the use of the bath, as it must wholly depend on the nature of the disease. The time allotted in the General Hospital is about three months; still in many slight disorders less time may be sufficient, but in paralytic cases and obstinate chronic disorders, and long-continued glandular obstructions, a much longer period than even three months is requisite.

In the use of the bath it is not necessary that any interruption should take place, as is the case with drinking the waters; indeed, in some disorders, particularly those of paralysis arising from mineral impregnations, I have known the bathing and pumping continued for six months with the most evident advantage, the limbs acquiring strength and motion, and the patient gradually recovering from his cadaverous appearance.

It should likewise be considered, that the majority of chronic cases sent to Bath are those in which every other remedy has been tried at a distance without success, and they are merely sent here as a forlorn hope; these cases are very discouraging, and frequently a perseverance during months is necessary, before the disorder begins to amend. This circumstance considered must make the cures in the General Hospital much more striking; for in many respects it may be deemed the hospital for incurables, none being sent here that could get relief by other means.

The other general directions necessary to enforce in the use of the baths are, moderate and regular exercise, great attention to the bowels, and abstinence from rich, high-seasoned, or stimulating food. The same observations, in these particulars, will hold good, as directed under the internal use of the waters. Many even of the local diseases have their origin in luxurious habits. To such we should say, pursue a contrary system; to those who suffer from the effects of climate, great debility, or accidental causes, more latitude may be allowed; but all must depend on the nature of the malady and the advice of the physician.

The opinion of Antonius Guainerius on the subject of hot baths may be here given, not on account of his direction to remain in the bath until the fingers begin to shrivel, which is rather an equivocal mode of judging; but because the latter part of his observations carry so much sound doctrine and good sense in them, that it would be an injury to alter his own language:

"*Semper in balneo tanta sit mora, quantum eum*
"*ibi stare delectat; vel donec digitorum pulpæ in*
"*rugis contractæ fuerint, ceteris tamen paribus*
"*longius mane, quam sero balneis immorandum*
"*erit. Cunque ab eis egreditur lectum intret, et*
"*ne a frigido tangatur aere se pānis cooperiat,*

"*dehinc in lecto sudorem tollerit, et cum minuere*
"*tamen perceperit, abstergatur, se postea induat et*
"*per aerem aliquantulum distantem a balneo per*
"*morulam ambulet; successive vero cibum boni*
"*chymi aut nutrimenti et facilis digestionis reci-*
"*piat, ab immoderato tamen cibi et potûs usu, et*
"*ab aliis hujusmodi se custodiat, et a coitu quam*
"*maxime.*"

With regard to the time of year most proper for bathing, we cannot do better than quote Dr. Lucas. "In fact, such is the temperature of our climate, "that we may use our warm baths, properly at-"tempered, in all the ordinary extremes of wea-"ther; but they must be found less dangerous in "the administering, as well as more efficacious, "during summer."

The above author likewise suggested the propriety of establishing a set of cold baths, where, after a course of hot bathing, the patients might strengthen themselves against the external cold by frequent immersions, before they return to their respective homes. This, however, appears superfluous.

In alluding to the benefit derived from the external application of the Bath waters, Dr. Saunders supposes that any water heated to the same temperature, and similarly applied, would produce similar effects. He judges and determines, from their chemical investigation, that the active ingredients are much too minute to exercise any stimulant power on the skin; that they can produce no other effect than common warm water; and that the invigorating properties ascribed to them must be erroneous.

This assertion in theory may be good, but facts are stubborn things; and a very little experience would convince the Doctor that the external application of the Bath water does not produce that relaxation and faintness experienced in common water; but, on the contrary, the patient feels his spirits lighter, and his whole frame invigorated and refreshed. He is able to continue in the bath a much longer period without distress; and many patients who came from a distant part of the country have tried common warm water bathing without success, previous to their determination to visit Bath.

The Doctor's evidence in favour of their virtues somehow or other escapes afterwards, notwithstanding his objections. He says, "it is the very "minute portions of active ingredients, so beauti- "fully arranged by that great chemist Nature, "which in reality produces their beneficial effects, "both internal and *external.*"

"In our baths," says Dr. Sutherland, "there "is a certain volatile principle, which (like elec- "trical æther) animates the whole man. Thus "bathing and drinking united exert their joint

" forces in opening obstructions, and promoting " secretions of every sort."

" The Bath waters externally used," observes Dr. Falconer, " are more stimulant than common " water. Sudden sweats and faintness, which often " come on after using a bath of common water of a " considerable degree of heat, rarely come on after " the use of the Bath waters; but the bathers are " observed to be in general more alert and vigorous, " and to have a better appetite, on the days of " bathing than in the intervals."

How the warm bath acts, is not to our present purpose to consider; that it does not relax, but rather invigorates, is clearly proved by the refreshment which is felt in bathing after violent fatigue, travelling, &c.; and it is well known that many of the hospital paralytics stay in more than an hour, in a temperature of upwards of 104°, which heat would evidently produce languor and debility, if the water did not possess some medicinal powers acting on the absorbents, and counteracting those debilitating effects, which would certainly proceed from common water heated to the same temperature.

It is the fashion with some sceptics to deny the power of the absorbents to imbibe any active principle from thermal waters. They may as well deny the action of sea water on the surface of the the body being different from common water;

they may go a step further, and deny the existence of absorbents at all, at least what in the general acceptation of the schools we call absorbents, they may as well deny the power of turpentine, which, rubbed on the surface, will produce effects on the secretions in the shortest period; of mercury producing salivation, of laudanum procuring sleep, and these acting entirely by external application; the absorption of the poison of venomous animals, of small-pox, cow-pox, &c. &c.

These instances have been dilated upon rather more fully, as I have heard very ingenious, sensible men deny the existence of absorbents altogether; and in illustration of the virtues of the Bath waters, it is very necessary to point out, that the benefit of their external application does not wholly arise from their increase of temperature, but principally from their medicinal impregnations.

Although many patients, from the nature of their complaints, and a natural timidity, prefer a private bath to the public; yet I am convinced much more benefit is to be derived from the latter; and in opposition to the opinion of many writers on the subject, we consider the public bath being open one of its strongest recommendations. Its exposure prevents an accumulation of confined steam and noxious vapours, which, it has been asserted, arises from a number of people bathing together, though the numbers are never sufficiently numerous to produce those bad consequences suggested by Dr. Lucas. Every patient will subscribe to the comfort and advantage of an open bath, who, during dry-pumping, has been enveloped in such a cloud of steam that he could not even see his own hand, and has felt the distressing head-ache which arises from the confined vapour. This, in my opinion, has frequently been a serious objection to the dry-pumping.

Some authors object to the open bath on the principle of the head being exposed, and the body heated, by which means a greater quantity of blood is forced up into the head, occasioning vertigos, apoplexies, &c. We can only speak from experience, that it does not produce those effects; and surely, according to correctness of logical reasoning, the head being kept cool would tend to relieve any disposition to plethora much more effectually than being smothered in the steam of the hot springs.

It is owing to the bath being open that I conceive paralytic patients suffer so little in the head from the use of bathing; for it is proved, contrary to the opinion of Dr. Meade, that paralysis is constantly benefited by its use; and in no instance, in the annals of the Bath Hospital, has apoplexy or hemiplegia arisen from this cause."

Dr. Falconer very justly observes, "we should "also consider that the patients are able to bear

" without faintness a greater degree of heat in an " open bath, than in one that is confined in a room."

The great advantage of a large open space must be very evident, when we consider the diseases for which the baths are principally advised. They are commonly affections of the joints, loss of action in the muscles, want of regular circulation, &c. all which diseases must be most materially benefited by constant exercise in the bath.

When it is also known that near a tun of water is discharged from the springs of the King's Bath every minute, and of course the same quantity carried off, what reason is there for the appellation of " uncleanliness and dirty water," &c. as applied to the public bath? The public bath possesses a thousand advantages not to be derived from the private ones; the first great advantage, as before stated, is being open and exposed to the heavens; the second is its natural discharge from the springs, and continual fresh supply; another desideratum is the size of the bath, where patients can walk about in a large volume of water of an equal temperature, for the quantity and heat of the bath is too great to be acted upon by the stones or sides of the bath. These once heated by such a body of water will always continue the same, although that has been a great objection to an open bath. The variation between the sides and centre of the bath is not half a degree, excepting immediately where the springs rise. The private bath must feel this objection tenfold; though the patient may go in at 96°, yet the moving about in so small a body of water will lessen the heat two degrees in two minutes, unless replenished with hot water, which I generally advise.

Our baths are by the invidious always compared and brought into competition with the Roman baths. Undoubtedly the latter were more elegant, and upon a much more extravagant scale; yet, from what we know of the Roman baths, they were mostly open. Even their forums, their theatres, were all open: the reason is evident—for the purpose of carrying off the exhalations and unpleasant effluvia excited by such an immense concourse of spectators as usually assembled on those occasions. It is upon the same principle our own baths are exposed; for added to the effluvia arising from the bathers, as very much exaggerated, the steam from the bath would most probably, if pent up without ventilation, do the patient more injury than the bathing confer benefit.

Though we consider the objection to the open bath as too insignificant to merit further observation, yet on one point there certainly may be some objections, viz. on the score of delicacy. I allude to the promiscuous bathing of the sexes, which the immense supply of water would fully enable the guardians of our hot springs to abolish.

We know from experience, that it is the wish, and has been the object for many years past, to render the accommodations both of drinking and bathing as commodious to the invalid as possible; and every suggestion for that purpose has been acted upon in the most liberal manner. Indeed, this very subject underwent considerable discussion a few years since, and alternate days were then appropriated for the bathing of ladies and gentlemen. The public, however, objected to the measure from a dislike to innovations, and not having the public baths at command every day as usual. The consequence was, after a few months' trial, the old system was restored. I am, notwithstanding, inclined to think, if a similar trial was again made, less objection would be raised, and a little time would conquer local prejudices.

Let us hear what the ancients thought of this custom, and see how far the encomium is applicable to the matrons and virgins of Bath.* "*Quod* "*autem scripsit Cassiodorus de aquis specialiter* "*fontis Aponi quòd temperaturam earum factum* "*pro viris, in qua balnearentur utilitur, fœminæ* "*tolerare non possent; ideo divulgatum, et credi*-"*tum antiquitas puto, quia temporibus illis nostræ* "*matronæ et virgines Patavinæ summa pudicitiæ* "*et verecundiæ gloria præstantes erant. Idque* "*per totam Italiam ita notum fuit, ut Valerialius*

Joannes de Doudis de aquis Patavinis, 107.

"*Martialis poeta, qui floruit sub imperio Domi-*
"*tiani, ideo dixerit,*

'*Fontes Aponi rudes puellis.*'

"*Hoc est intactos, et non aditos ab illis, quia propter honestatem et verecundiam non ingrederentur in ea balnea; et non propter fervorem qui eis possit nocere, in quibus viri balnearentur; cum tamen in aliis locis et urbibus non esset ista verecundia et honestas, sed mulieres promiscue cum viris lavarentur, quod patet de Romanis apud poetas; et tanta fuit fama pudicitiæ nostrarum Matronarum, ut Martialis supradictus, cum vellet fæminam pudicissiman dicere, Patavinam dixerit, notissimo illo versu,* 'SIS PATAVINA LICET.'

"*Ego autem frequenter vidi sine aliqua læsione in virorum balneis, fæminas balneari; et, quod pro pudor, multo impudentius est, vidi etiam simul aliquando mares et fæminas in eodem balneo; est tamen procul dubio verum quod magis ferventem aquam, et calidiorem temperaturam possunt tolerare mares, quàm fæminæ, non solum aquæ fontis Aponi, et aliarum thermarum, sed etiam dulcium balneorum, propter soliditatem majorem carnium, et cutium virorum quàm fæminarum.*"

From every inquiry I was able to make at the time, I could not understand that the objection was raised by any real invalids; but principally by those who certainly wished to bathe, but who would not allow it to interfere with the balls, the theatre, or bad weather. Those were the only arguments I could ever hear advanced; and although fewer people resorted to the bath, yet there had not been sufficient time for the new regulations to be known, and the consequence was repeated disappointments. Waving, however, any speculations as to whether the public would like to be deprived of the option of bathing when they please, we may be allowed to make a suggestion, which would reconcile all contending opinions.

The object is to prove that the supply of water from the spring at the King's Bath is amply sufficient to form two baths, both to be filled in as short a period as the Cross Bath now is; one for the accommodation of the ladies, the other for the gentlemen.

The King's Bath at present is 66 feet in length, and 41 feet in breadth, and the Queen's Bath 25 feet square, filling in eleven hours. The grand object I conceive for the accommodation of the public would be the enlargement of the King's Bath, and so dividing it as to make a good-sized bath for the daily use of both the ladies and the gentlemen. This might easily be accomplished by the extension of the King's Bath on the south side, making it 66 feet square, or even larger, if it were thought necessary. A slight ashler partition, about seven feet high, might be thrown over the centre of the bath, in the form of an arch, three feet deep, to allow both sides of the partition to be of the same temperature, and filled at the same time. This would form two handsome baths, one for gentlemen and one for ladies, each 66 feet long by 33 feet wide. The idea of the arched partition is to prevent the weight of a wall from pressing on the springs, and to allow the communication of the water at the same time.

I am aware that an extension of the King's Bath on the south side would encroach on the Queen's Bath, which lies to the south of the King's, and that it would actually take in part of the Queen's Bath. The vacant ground, however, on the south of the Queen's Bath would, under this arrangement, be appropriated to form part of a new Queen's Bath; which would be the principal alteration, and might be effected at a very trifling expense. With regard to the supply of water, which is another consideration:—supposing the King's and Queen's Baths were both enlarged one-half beyond their present dimensions, the present supply of water is sufficient to fill them in sixteen hours and a half, being less time than is required to fill the Cross Bath. The addition, however, now suggested would not take more than two hours or two hours and a half.

One great advantage in this plan is, that it would give not the least interruption to bathers whilst in progress. The only difference would be, that bathers who require a temperate bath would go to the Cross Bath, as the Queen's Bath must of course be shut out from the King's, and every preparation outside might be made, till they were ready to be united.

With regard to an enlargement of the Queen's Bath, that is not necessary, 25 feet square being quite sufficient. The heat of the Queen's Bath is 96°, and the heat of the Cross Bath varies very little from that temperature, or it might, indeed, be exactly the same; thus the public have already two large open baths of the same heat, one of which might be considered the ladies' and the other the gentlemen's bath, for one of these baths at present is quite superfluous.

If the improvements here stated could be carried into effect, many advantages would accrue to the patient which are now overlooked, because they cannot be remedied. I allude to the cumbrous dresses which are at present worn by those who frequent the public baths. Dresses of any kind very much defeat the intention, by preventing the water from coming immediately in contact with those parts of the body which are the situations of disease. If the patients could bathe without being encumbered with a dress at all, it would be most eligible; but if a dress must be worn, it should be as light and loose as possible; and the advantage of separate baths for men and women would greatly promote this intention.

The assertions of Dr. Lucas and others against open baths and promiscuous bathing is by no means correct. At Baden in Switzerland, Baden, near Vienna, Buda in Hungary, and even Borcet, near Aix-la-Chapelle, the baths are all open, and the sexes bathe promiscuously. This we do not mention by way of justification, but only to remove an impression that "Bath is the only place where such "scandalous abuses exist."

Now we are on the subject of improvements, it may not be amiss to suggest the propriety of stoves being substituted in the anti-rooms to the private baths in lieu of fire-places. Too great a fire in warm weather is very apt to produce perspiration, and consequent relaxation after coming out of the bath, and dispose the patient to take cold. This is no suppositious case, but one frequently complained of. Abroad they have no open fire-places, but stoves so regulated as not to be oppressive in warm weather.

Having thus stated in general terms the diseases for which the hot baths are particularly recommended; having also given an account of the various baths, their temperature, and mode of application; and having taken the liberty of suggesting such improvements as would, in our opinion, elevate the thermal arrangements to the highest pitch of excellence; we shall now retrogade a little, and compare the poor and miserable accommodations which the baths afforded to invalids in former times, with the superior conveniences of the present day.

Leland gives a very wretched description of the baths in his Itinerary. At this time they were rented by the Corporation; but one great bar to their improvement was, that they hardly possessed an inch of ground beyond the baths, which prevented their extension, or making those accommodations which since have been so liberally accomplished. Private property at this time extended close to the baths; the houses adjoining generally were lodging-houses, kept by the physicians, and had openings directly communicating with the baths. This was undoubtedly a private benefit, but it likewise became a private source of emolument and competition, much to the detriment of the public. As for public accommodations, there was not so much as a hovel, even by the King's Bath, wherein a guide or poor person could deposit his clothes while in the bath, and they were obliged to leave them in the common entrance, till a cabin was made for that purpose.

So late as the reign of Elizabeth few people did more than bathe, there being no certainty of the water being pure. It was in this reign the Corporation were made perpetual guardians of the city and the hot waters, and from this period we may date the improvements that took place in our public baths, as the Corporation previously had very little interest, and certainly no power to rectify the abuses so much complained of.

Indeed, it was many years before these abuses could be rectified, and not until the Corporation obtained considerable extension both of their power and property. It was at this period that the baths are represented as like so many bear gardens, every kind of filth being thrown into them, every indecency practised; smoking tobacco, singing songs, and making other disturbances, to the annoyance of the invalid, and the total subversion of good government in the city. These disorders proceeded to such a pitch, that a memorial was drawn up and presented to James I.; but that monarch dying, nothing was determined in consequence. Some years afterwards some regulations were resolved upon, which had the good effect of remedying these abuses; and from one improvement to another, the baths are at present as commodious as any in this kingdom.

The practice of bathing has fallen very much into disuse amongst the modern nations of Europe. Amongst the ancients the baths were public buildings, under the immediate cognizance of the government; they were, literally speaking, the physic of the age; with very little assistance the bath was the remedy for every disease. The fable of Medea boiling people to restore youth was no doubt metaphorically meant to signify the benefit experienced from warm bathing, or immersion in hot mineral springs. Among the Turks, bathing forms a part of actual existence; and in every village is a bath for the benefit of the public. The Egyptians, likewise, consider bathing not merely as a luxury, but one of the necessaries of life. From the Greeks, who carried bathing to an excess little short of the Romans, the latter have derived their term *thermæ*. "*Græci fontes aquarum calidarum* θερμὰς *appellant.*" The vapour baths in Russia have been celebrated from time immemorial; thus we may trace the antiquity of bathing originally to the eastern nations, from thence to the Greeks, and from the latter to the Romans.

It is well known that the baths at Rome, of which near eight hundred existed at one time, were not merely used medicinally, but considered the greatest luxury; in which the common people indulged; and which ultimately was carried to such a pitch of extravagance and licentiousness, that several imperial decrees were necessary to repress its destructive excess.

The magnificent ruins of the baths of Titus and Caracalla, also the remains of the baths of Constantine, are visible proofs of the grandeur of design and execution effected in those days; but amongst the noblest monuments of ancient Rome were reckoned the thermæ or baths of Dioclesian; and to shew the stupendous undertakings of the Romans, it is only necessary to mention that in the great hall of the baths of Dioclesian, which was converted into a church by Michael Angelo, the granite columns, which are still preserved, are *single stones*, each forty feet in height.

Although the Romans carried their bathing at a later period to the most pernicious excess, and decency and morality were alike disregarded, yet in the purer state of society there were separate baths, both public and private, for the women as well as for the men; and that promiscuous bathing was not only forbidden, but unlawful, appears from the following passage extracted from Gesner *de Thermis Helveticis.* "*Viri et fœminæ balneis communibus utuntur: etsi leges sacræ et Canones infamem illum faciant qui cum mulieribus balneatur; quod si conjugem habuerit donationem propter nuptias perdat, et mulier alieno cum viro balneans, dotem perdit; ut cap. de repud. L. Junto. Lege cavetur Lombardica. Si vir thermas mulieribus discretas violenter intrare præsumpserit, capite puniatur. Nam Carthaginensis synodus conclusit non oportere altaris ministros, ullosve Christianos, lavacra habere communia. Legimus etiam a Julio Capitolino Historico, M. Aurelium Antoninum*

Imperatorem, collaudatum quæ lavacra mixta submovisset."

The finest specimens of baths in this country, after the model of the Roman baths, are those discovered in this city, which were undoubtedly built under the inspection of the Romans; and it is to be regretted that on the discovery of these beautiful remnants of antiquity the whole of the baths had not been excavated, and their foundations fairly traced. We might then have had the advantage of using the identical Roman baths so highly praised by Solinus; or even if the spring had been lost, or their site too low for present use, their preservation might have been secured by a walled fence, and they would have remained the delight of the antiquary, and an everlasting monument of the original grandeur of this elegant city.

The excavations of Herculaneum and Pompeii are considered as national works, and the honour of the country interested in their progress. Here we have a specimen of grandeur and magnificence which would do honour to Herculaneum, or even Rome herself, accidentally discovered in the highest state of preservation; and yet, with a Vandalism wholly unaccountable, they are buried amidst a chaos of filth to form the foundations of beggarly houses, that never can repay their elevation.

These baths, it is known, were discovered under the Priory, in the year 1755, and were then seen by Dr. Lucas, who conjectured that what was then visible was merely one wing of a magnificent building, and that further examination, if it were possible, would probably shew a corresponding wing on the western side, beyond the great bath. On some further examination taking place in 1799 and 1803, these ideas were found to be correct, and part of corresponding foundations were discovered, similar to the eastern wing. The lithographic etching shews the part of the baths discovered at various times, and their connexion will very easily be perceived. Although we have given an account of these baths in the History of Bath, extracted from Collinson's Somerset, yet, as a further illustration of a most interesting subject, we shall here add Dr. Lucas's account:

"Under the foundation of the Abbey House, "full ten feet deep, appear traces of a bath, whose "dimensions are 43 feet by 34. Within, and ad-"joining to the walls, are the remains of twelve "pilasters, each measuring three feet six inches "on the front of the plinth, by a projection of "two feet three inches. These pillars seem to "have supported a roof. This bath stood north "and south.

"To the northward of this room, parted only "by a slender wall, with an opening of about ten "inches in the middle, adjoined a semicircular bath, "measuring from east to west 14 feet 4 inches, and

" from the crown of the semicircle to the partition " wall which divides it from the square bath, 18 feet " 10 inches. The roof of this seems to have been " sustained by four pilasters, one at each angle, and " two at the springing of the circle. This bath " seems to have undergone some alteration, the " base of the semicircle is filled up to about the " height of five feet, upon which two pilasters were " set on either side from the area, between two " separate flights of steps, into the semicircular part, " which seems to be all that was reserved for a " bath. In this was placed a stone chair, eighteen " inches high and sixteen broad. The two flights " of steps were of different dimensions: those to " the west were three feet nine inches broad, those " to the east four feet two inches. Each flight " consists of steps six inches thick, and seems to " have been worn by use three inches and a half " out of the square. These flights are divided by " a stone partition, on a level with the floor. " Along this division, and along the west side of " the area, a rude channel, of about three inches " depth, was cut in the stone. The floor of this " bath seems to be on a level with that of the " square bath.

" Eastward from the area and stairs of the " semicircular bath, stood an elegant room on each " side, sustained by four pilasters.

" Separated by a wall stood the *Hypocausta* " *Laconica*, or *stoves*, to the eastward. These " consisted of two large rooms, each measuring 39 " feet by 22; each had a double floor, one of " which lay one foot nine inches lower than the " area round the square bath. On this lower floor " stand rows of pillars, composed of square bricks, " of about an inch and three quarters thick, and " nine inches square. These pillars sustain a " second floor, composed of tiles two feet square, " and two inches thick, over which are laid two " layers of firm cement mortar, each about two " inches thick, which compose the upper floor.

" To the northward, separated by a wall of three " feet eleven inches, stood the other *Hypocaus-* " *tum*, with a door of communication. The floor " of this is about eighteen inches higher than the " other.

" These two rooms are set round with square " brick *tubes* of different lengths, from sixteen to " twenty inches in length, and six and three quar- " ters wide. These flues have two lateral openings, " of about two inches square, five inches asunder. " These open into the vacuum between these two " floors, and rise through the walls. The north " wall of the last stove was filled with tubes of a " lesser size, placed horizontally and perpendicu- " larly. The stones and bricks between the pillars " bear evident marks of fire, while the flues are

" strongly charged with soot, which plainly point " out their uses.

" Heat was communicated to these flues by " means of *præfurnia*. In the middle of the " northern wall of the second stove, the ruins of " one of these furnaces appear. It consists of " strong walls of about sixteen feet square, with an " opening in the centre of about three feet wide, " which terminates conically in the north wall of " the stove, two feet wide, where part of the " broken arch bears evident marks of fire. About " the mouth of the furnace there were scattered " pieces of burnt wood, charcoal, &c. evident " proofs of their use.

" On each side of the furnace, adjoining to the " wall of the northermost stove, is a semicircular " chamber, of about ten feet four inches by nine " feet six. Their floors are nearly two feet six " inches lower than that of the next stove, into " which they both open. The pavements are tes- " selated with variegated rows of pebbles and red " bricks.

" To the northward of these appear ruins of two " other square chambers, of more ordinary work."

In Dr. Jones's map of the city of Bath there is a tennis-court adjoining the bath, 81 feet by 27, with a private door to open into the bath for the accommodation of the players. This appears to be an imitation of the Roman gymnasia; for to the

Roman thermæ was united every institution which could afford exercise to the body, or relaxation to the mind.

Thus we have given a statement of these noble baths, as described by Dr. Lucas, and have only to repeat our regret that the baths were not pursued to their full extent. There are many reasons for wishing such had been the case, for on a review of the baths it will be perceived, that, beside the private baths and sudatories, in the *one wing alone there is a public bath*, 41 *feet by* 34; in the western wing similar accommodations, and *another public bath*, 41 *feet by* 34; and in the centre, *the grand public bath*, 90 *feet by* 68. Let us pause a little, examine the dimensions of these baths, and then enquire where is the spring which is to renew them daily, as undoubtedly was the case at the period of their erection? That the spring exists at this moment in the centre of the grand public bath, I have no more doubt than I have of the existence of the baths themselves; and if the excavations had been properly pursued, there would it have been found. All our springs together are not sufficient for the supply of baths of such magnitude. Would the Romans, who studied convenience as well as elegance in all their buildings, have erected baths at a distance from the springs? Certainly not. *They built upon the springs*, that they might flow, with as little diminution of heat as possible, to supply the grand bath first, then the smaller public baths, and the private baths. Look at the situation of the King's Bath, compare it with the centre of the Roman bath; I do not believe they have the slightest communication. The King's is a spring of itself, as is demonstrated by its great heat; if it filtered through the earth from the Roman bath, and was a part of that spring, it certainly would be diminished in temperature, and occasionally in quantity.

II. On Pumping.

Pumping being advised in two different ways, has usually been denominated wet and dry pumping; the former from being used whilst in the warm bath, the latter applied locally on the limb or part affected without immersion. These various applications of the pump have been deservedly ranked amongst the most effectual means of relief in local disorders.

The origin of wet and dry pumping may be traced to Dr. Jorden, at whose instigation regular pumps were erected; thus he promoted and improved the external application of the waters, although he would not recommend their internal use. Prior to the Doctor's practising at Bath, *bucketing*, or the *douse*, was the mode commonly used; which was thus performed: two of the tallest and strongest of the guides stood with the patient in the hottest part of the bath, and lifting up a full bucket as high as they could, they then let the water fall leisurely upon the part affected. But the Doctor finding this method did not heat some sufficiently, he caused pumps to be erected to draw it as hot as possible from the spring. Four of these pumps were erected in the four principal baths, in recesses made for that purpose, and called wet pumps; and one was placed in a little room, built over part of a slip at the end of the Hot Bath, and named the dry pump, as not communicating with the bath.

The mode of external bathing used by the Romans was similar to the *douse*; "the water was "taken up and poured on the head and particular "parts from pitchers and urns, from greater or "lesser heights. In some cases the bathers came "out of the hot water, were anointed, and re-"turned. In others they did not go into the "water, but sat down by the side of the bath, and "had the water poured on them."

The water from the pump falls from a perpendicular height of 14 feet, which is fully sufficient for every medicinal purpose, as in many instances the patient is hardly able to bear even this column of water. At Paris, at the artificial baths, the highest *douche* falls from a height of 32 French feet.

At the present day there are pumps connected with all the baths, both public and private; and two dry pumps, with dressing-rooms adjoining, and every conveniency, one at the King's Bath, and the other at the Hot Bath.

Various are the diseases in which pumping is recommended as an auxiliary to the bath; and in some local affections pumping without the bath proves of the greatest service. In rigidity, contractions of the joints, indolent tumours, gouty, rheumatic, and paralytic limbs, luxations, sprains, debility from local injuries, such as fractures, &c. and almost every species of local disease, unattended by inflammation. The pump is very much recommended in all local affections arising from want of circulation, and applied to the different parts of the body, as the head,* neck, spine, or limbs, as the seat of the disorder may point out. Pumping on the spine has been found most serviceable in diseases connected with the uterus, in local weaknesses, obstinate pains, &c.

The mode of using the pump, as already observed, is either in the bath or out of it. When

* Though pumping on the head has been recommended by many authors, yet I think the pumping of the Bath waters on the head is rather an objectionable practice. I am convinced I have seen it do injury.

used in the bath it appears to give a general warmth and pleasing sensation, but its force is not particularly felt; neither do we think it of that benefit in relieving pain, or promoting circulation, which is evidently experienced by the dry pumping. It is, however, very useful in cases of extreme debility, and to patients of delicate temperament, who are unable to bear the extraordinary force of the other pump.

It is the external application, or the dry pump, which we more particularly recommend, and which will be found one of the most effectual remedies in the relief afforded to old chronic pains or lamenesses, which probably for years have resisted every other application. The heat of the pump cannot be modified; it is poured on the afflicted part of the patient by means of a flexible tube communicating with the pump and reservoir on the outside, and when first pumped on the limb, appears almost scalding hot, and with very great force. This feeling, however, soon subsides, and after the proper number of strokes, the surface of the part appears red and inflamed, with a glowing sensation, for some time.

The pump, though discharged in a continued stream, is nevertheless measured by the number of strokes or elevation of the handle of the pump, used by the assistant. It is customary to begin with 50 or 100 strokes, and to increase the number according to the nature of the case and ability of the patient to bear it. Formerly patients were ordered from one to two thousand strokes, but our more moderate practice generally confines it to three or four hundred. The usual charge is threepence a hundred in the bath, and sixpence a hundred out of it. This consideration has preserved the mode of directing the pump by the number; but it would certainly appear more correct to direct its application by the time, five, ten, or fifteen minutes, and charge accordingly.

When bathing is directed at the same time as the pumping, they may be used on alternate days; if the dry pumping be recommended alone, there is no objection to its use every day; but if by its perseverance a degree of inflammation and eruption should appear on the surface of the skin, it had better be omitted a few days, until these symptoms have disappeared, and then be resumed.

After using the pump, the patient should keep the limb moderately warm, and walk as usual Indeed, it must be apparent, that in all rigidities, lameness, or want of circulation, regular exercise will materially assist the benefit to be expected from the application of the pump.

The preparation necessary for the pump is exactly similar to the directions for drinking and bathing. It is more than probable that many of the local diseases originate from constitutional predisposition, most certainly gout and many others ; and it would be very unwise to use every local means for the recovery of the effects, and neglect those means which would strike at the cause.

The cases generally recommended for the pump are most commonly those of very long standing, which have tried almost every other application before they have been sent here. In consequence, it is very difficult to state the exact time patients should remain; I think this point should be decided by the benefit they receive. It is, however, too often the case, that as soon as a little amendment is perceived, the patient runs away, when a continuance of the plan would probably effect a cure.

When the object is to recover a limb, or remove a disease which may prove a torment as long as we live, no sacrifice can be too dear. And where money and time are no object, the best plan is, to take a house for a twelvemonth, with a fixed determination to devote that time to the recovery of health. Such resolution will in the end be amply repaid.

With regard to medical means, whether any and what would be proper, must be entirely omitted in this place. As we have recommended the pumping for a variety of diseases, so each disease must have its discretionary treatment, which no general rules can possibly direct. One observation will, however, apply to this, and indeed every other deviation from health,—to keep the mind easy, the bowels open, take regular and moderate exercise without fatigue, and live a stemiously.

III. On the Vapour Bath.

The vapour bath or sudatory is situated at the Hot Bath, and can be graduated to any temperature. It is accommodated with a dressing-room and other conveniences; it is, however, one of the least convenient of the thermal arrangements in this city, and not applicable as a local remedy.

It is probably owing to the admirable accommodations for bathing and pumping, and the diseases for which the sudatory is recommended being similar, which in some degree prevents the more frequent application of the steam bath. It is a remedy, however, which amongst the ancients was in the highest degree of estimation, being regarded not only medicinally, but as one of the greatest luxuries, and which was invariably attached to the Roman thermæ, under the appellation of the *Laconicum*.

It appears the Romans divided their sudatories into two species, the dry and the moist; the one, hot vapour, or the *Laconicum;* the other, hot air introduced into rooms, called *Hypocausta*, *Stuphæ*, or stoves.

The *Laconicum* was round, concamerated, filled with hot vapour from the subjacent furnace, as well as the steam of hot water. Here persons sweated profusely. From the *Laconicum*, the bather went into the *Calidarium*, or warm water bath, and from thence directly plunged into the *Frigidarium*, or cold bath.

The *Hypocausta*, or *Stuphæ*, were hot apartments; the heat was conducted through tubes, and under the floors, and within the walls, the vapour exhaling through every part of the building. The ancient Germans conducted the heat from a furnace through various tubes into ornaments, figures, or statues, which poured forth hot air insensibly through their nostrils, ears, eyes, spears, &c.

The vapour bath is particularly serviceable in softening and relaxing the fibres, cleansing and opening the pores, curing herpetic and all cutaneous eruptions, promoting perspiration, easing pains, cramps, contractions, and rigidity of limbs and joints, in relieving paralytic and gouty affections, together with all chronic rheumatism, such as sciatica, lumbago, &c. and in dispersing ædematous tumours. It is also particularly useful in relaxing uterine constrictions, and removing obstructions, and promoting a more regular and equal circulation in those parts where it had previously been extremely languid.

The time for using the vapour bath should certainly be early in the morning, on an empty stomach; but where it is recommended for the removal of obstructions in the pores arising from cold, or from eruptive diseases suddenly disappearing, of course any time may then be chosen, as the disease must have immediate relief. How long it should be continued, and how often repeated, must depend on the continuance of the disease.

Dr. Kentish, who has paid the greatest attention to this branch of science, recommends it as a most efficacious and decided remedy in many disorders, where it is properly applied. Mr. La Baume has also published some cases in which its powers are strongly depicted.

The Hon. Basil Cochrane has spent many years, and been at considerable expense, in bringing to perfection the vapour bath, and for simplicity and efficiency his apparatus appears by far the best.

Mr. Cochrane observes, "in all chronic affec-"tions it has seldom failed to give immediate relief, "and if persevered in, of performing a perfect "cure. Severe paroxysms of the gout and rheu-"matism, contractions of the joints, and obstinate "humours, have readily yielded to its powers. In "colds and pains of the chest it is particularly "efficacious, and head-aches and the tooth-ache are "almost always considerably mitigated, and often "totally dispelled by it. Hence it is demonstrable, "that the vapour bath is one of the most essential "requisites in every family for the purposes of "health; and it may also be used in the comforts of "ablution, and applied to the purposes of luxury."

According to Mr. Cochrane's plan, vapour of any degree of heat may be applied generally, or to any individual part of the body, and medicated if required. He also recommends the Russian practice of flagellating with twigs, or shampooing according to the Eastern fashion, after quitting the bath.

His plan of a portable steam bath was, placing a boiler on a common fire, with a flexible tube to communicate with the bath, and a stop cock to regulate the heat. If a medicated bath were required, the flexible tube screwed on to a pewter vessel, in which herbs, &c. were placed, and through which the hot air is passed. In the same way the regulated heat might be conveyed by the tube under the bed-clothes to a patient unable to sit or lay down on the frame-work of the bath. By means of this tube, with a funnel-shaped top to screw on, it is easy to conceive how the vapour may be applied topically, without exposing the whole body to the action of the steam.

The Russian sudatories are conducted in the following manner. In the bath room is a large vaulted oven, which, when heated, makes the paving-stones lying upon it red hot. Round about the walls are three or four rows of benches, one above another like the seats of a scaffold. The room has little light, but apertures to let the vapour escape, the cold water that is wanted being let in by small channels. The heat in the bath-room is usually from 32° to 40° of Reaumur, and this is much increased by throwing water every five minutes on the glowing hot stones in the chamber of the oven. Thus the heat often rises to 44° of Reaumur. The persons that bathe lie quite naked on one of the benches, when they perspire, more or less, in proportion to the heat of the humid atmosphere in which they are enveloped. For promoting perspiration, and more completely opening the pores, they are first rubbed, and then gently flagellated with leafy bunches of birch. After remaining for some time in this state, they come down from the sweating bench, and wash their bodies with warm or cold water, and at last plunge over head in a large tub of water. Many persons throw themselves immediately from the bath-room into the adjoining river, or roll themselves in the snow.*

A sweating bath similar to the above might very easily be made in any private house. A brick flue carried round a room, and well heated, and a strong frame-work of cane or whipcord suspended above the flue for the patients to lie on. The

* Tooke's View of the Russian Empire.

doors should be well closed, so as not to admit the air, and a small pipe of water immediately above the flue and under the frame-work, with holes at the under part of the pipe, so that when the cock is turned, the water may fall equally on every part of the hot flue, and the vapour ascend in every direction. The efficacy of this bath would depend on the heat of the brick, which must be made very hot, or sufficient steam will not arise.

The length of time for the use of the vapour-bath is from five to twenty minutes; but if it occasion much flushing in the face, or uneasiness in the head, it must be omitted. After the steam-bath the patient should lie down on a sofa for half an hour and be well rubbed, before venturing home.

The other medical directions should be rigidly observed, as pointed out under the chapters on bathing and pumping; but as the patient should by no means use the vapour-bath without medical advice, further directions on these points are unnecessary.

We cannot quit this subject without again remarking, that the vapour-bath, *of proper construction*, and judiciously applied, is one of the most powerful remedies in a variety of formidable complaints; and we have no doubt, that in a very short time its penetrating virtues will be duly appreciated.

Since writing the above, I have been favoured with an inspection of the portable vapour bath, improved by Mr. Moody, and for which he has obtained a patent. It has the advantage of great simplicity, and easy application; and the regulation of the temperature can, with the est ease, be directed by the patient himself. His other vapour-baths for the application of vapour to any particular part, should be the model for those erected at the Hot Bath. On the whole we consider the patent portable vapour-bath a grand desideratum amongst our medicinal resources; and its application is so simple, and its beneficial effects so decided in a multitude of disorders arising from checked perspiration, that we shall expect to hail the day when every private family will have a portable vapour machine as a necessary part of their establishment.

IV. The Shower Bath.

The Shower Bath is likewise situated at the Hot Bath, and has all the conveniences of the other baths. It may be directed of any heat, and likewise any quantity of water from one to fourteen gallons.

It is directed in a variety of complaints, but is not a remedy particularly illustrative of the beneficial effect of the Bath waters, as it is seldom ordered of the natural heat, but principally at a low temperature, preparatory to its cold application.

V. The Injecting Machine.

The Lavement, or Injecting Machine, is situated at the King's Bath, and was the invention of the late Morgan Nichols, esq; surgeon. There is likewise another at the Hot Bath, upon the same principle. To each a dressing-room and water-closet are attached.

The injection, which can be thrown up with very great force, is acted upon by the pressure of the reservoir above, which is filled with water from the hot springs; and moderated in its strength by moving a spring at the side of the machine. This can be regulated by the patients themselves, according to their ability to endure its force.

This machine is not recommended by any specific virtue of the waters; for the Bath waters in this case are only of service as always affording a proper medium of temperature, and a constant supply for the employment of its mechanical powers.

We know of no remedy which has proved of so much advantage, or afforded relief from the most imminent danger, comparable with the injection bath; the ease with which it is administered, the force with which it is injected, and the invariable supply of the tepid fluid to renew its operations, render it one of the most pleasant as well as effectual means which can be directed for the removal of obstinate obstructions of the bowels.

Every practitioner must have witnessed distressing cases of this kind; where the most intense anxiety is excited to observe the operation of medicine; when we see dose after dose taken without effect, nausea coming on, tension of the bowels, inflammation rapidly advancing, and still no relief, and these symptoms increasing hourly; in such cases this machine, by steady perseverance, has been the means of rescuing many a valuable life, which, under other circumstances, must inevitably have been sacrificed.

Many cases might be related of recovery from situations where "death appeared staring the patient "in the face;" and others certainly more distressing, where, from organic disease, no relief could be obtained. I should, however, be very loth to consider a case as hopeless, till I had seen the use of the injection bath tried repeatedly without effect. The various cases in which I have seen it succeed and one particularly under my own roof) would always embolden me to expect a favourable result from its use, if unattended by organic affection.

Independent of its advantage in violent stages of constipation and inflammation, it is of the greatest use in paralytic disorders, where the action of the intestinal canal partakes of the nature of the disease. In such cases, where relief is obtained with the greatest difficulty, medicine often produces nausea at the stomach, with loss of appetite, fretfulness at the medicine not operating, (though very violent,) and a whole host of dyspeptic symptoms. To invalids labouring under these symptoms, (and very many such come to Bath,) the injection is the best remedy which can be devised. They can go every day, or every other day, at a certain hour, and after relief feel happy the rest of the day at not being dosed with physic, and being released from the disappointment and nausea usually attending its exhibition.

To other invalids who are distressed by a costive habit, or often by a want of proper stimulus in the rectum itself, the machine will be very beneficial; and if persevered in, may promote a more regular action, and relieve the torpor of the lower bowels.

In many cases of hemorrhoids, arising from confined state of the bowels, internal heat, or the exhibition of aloetic medicines, this machine, used regularly every other morning, has effected wonders.

It has not only removed the disease itself, but the tendency to it, and eventually brought on a regular state of the excretions.

As a general relief on all occasions, it is extremely useful; and one great recommendation may be, the knowledge that an alderman of this city, who died at a *good old age*, never dined at a civic feast without first paying his devotions at this inestimable altar; and to this grand remedy he attributed his almost uninterrupted good health.

VI. The Pediluvium.

The Pediluvium, or Foot Bath, is a remedy more frequently used at Bath than most other places, from the convenience of the hot springs, and from the deep tubs in which the water is conveyed, which reaches nearly to the knees.

In combination with other means, it is a very useful auxiliary in relieving obstructions, and promoting a more general circulation. The best time for using the foot bath is at bed-time, and the length of time from five to ten minutes. It generally produces a soothing pleasant sensation, encouraging perspiration and promoting sleep.

In some severe head-aches this remedy is very beneficial, particularly when the hands and feet are cold, and the circulation languid. If, however, the extremities are much heated, with face flushed, and throbbing of the temples, the pediluvium may do great injury by encouraging an increase of action which is already too great, and which should be relieved by medicine and bleeding, either topical or general.

This remedy is often very useful in assisting obstructed catamenia, and may be directed for several nights following, in conjunction with gentle aloetic medicines.

The ancients recommended bathing the feet for a variety of complaints; they also considered it an antidote to sterility; thus Gardano *de aquis fervidis.* "*Eo ipso in balneo saxum rotundum* "*est, in medio cavum satis profunde, in quo mu-* "*lieres steriles insertos pedes aliquandiu retinent,* "*hoc ad fœcunditatem eis facere persuasæ.*"

Though bathing the feet is considered one of those common remedies which every one may prescribe, yet where the use of it is designed not as a luxury, but for the removal or prevention of disease, an attention to the state of the *primæ viæ* should not be disregarded. Every remedy which may do good, by parity of reasoning may do harm, if injudiciously applied.

VII. The Hip Bath.

In stating the various modes of using the baths, we have thought it right to mention all the methods by which they can be possibly recommended. The Hip Bath is a local bath, something in the shape of a wheel-barrow.

This bath may be used of any temperature, and is principally directed in rheumatic cases, such as *lumbago* or *sciatica*, also in weaknesses of the loins or local pains, where it is not advisable for the patient to go into a regular bath.

The method of using it is for the patient to sit in the bath, by which means the upper and lower part of the body do not come in contact with the water, but it merely covers the seat of the disease.

Whatever benefit may be expected from the hip bath I think may be felt in a tenfold degree by the application of a local vapour bath; and there can be little doubt but the one will supersede the other, when it is better known and appreciated.

The medical means, in conjunction with the hip bath, must be directed by the medical adviser, as the bath can only be considered as part of a system in aid of some general plan of treatment.

The application of the Bath waters to the various stages of disease will come next under consideration; and to the view of the unjaundiced, unprejudiced observer, we trust it will be acknowledged, that the salutary effect of our medicinal springs in chronic distempers, is not exceeded by any remedy in the known world. For the evidence of our assertions we appeal to facts.

ON GOUT.

THE gout has usually been considered an hereditary disease, although it also affects persons without any such disposition; but it can generally be traced to a sedentary life, and indulgence in the luxuries of the table. It more frequently attacks males than females, and principally those of robust habits and irregular lives. Where, however, it arises from hereditary taint, the most abstemious may be subject to it. It is a disease which in different persons puts on such a variety of forms as to render its history very inadequate as a general description.

The gout is an inflammatory affection of some of the smaller joints, often coming on suddenly without any warning, but generally preceded by some disordered state of the stomach, as flatulency, indigestion, &c. which appears to subside on the advancement of the fit. Most gouty patients have, likewise, a disposition to gravel; and a common forerunner of a fit is high-coloured urine, depositing a strong brick-coloured sediment. It most commonly affects the first joint of the great toe, attended with redness and swelling of the part, and accompanied with slight shivering and feverish symptoms. It generally remits in twenty-four hours, by the coming on of a gentle sweat. The disease often continues in this way for some days, and then gradually subsides, not returning for a considerable period.

As the disease advances, its attacks are more frequent, and various joints become affected, removing suddenly from one part to another, and eventually affecting the larger joints likewise. The pain in these attacks is often excessive, the patient hardly being able to bear the weight of the bedclothes on the affected limb.

Although in the earlier stages of the gout very little stiffness is left after the departure of the fit; yet the frequent occurrence of the attacks at length produces great rigidity of the muscles, a thickening of the capsular ligament surrounding the joints, and a vitiated secretion of the synovial fluid with chalky deposits, which ultimately destroy motion altogether.

It very often, however, happens, that the gout does not go through this regular progress, but from constitutional or accidental causes either does not amount to a regular fit, or when proceeding in the regular way, the inflammation suddenly disappears, and produces morbid symptons in some vital part.

The first species of this irregular gout, termed the atonic gout, is, when there is every feeling of the disease in the constitution without inflammation of the joints, exciting nausea, vomiting, flatulency, acid eructations, and pains about the region of the stomach. These affections are also attended with an irregular state of the bowels, all the symptons of hypochondriasis, flying pains felt about the body, and the chest and head sometimes disordered.

The other species of this disease is termed the retrocedent gout. Thus when the gout comes on in the regular way, producing inflammation of the joints, &c. it suddenly recedes, and some internal part becomes immediately affected. If the affected part be the stomach, it is attended with anxiety, sickness, or violent pain; if the heart, syncope; if the lungs, asthma; and if the head, palsy or apoplexy. Gouty patients are also more or less subject to nephritic affections, arising from calculi in the kidneys; and these attacks frequently alternate with fits of the gout.

Though it is not our intention to enter into a long dissertation on this variable malady, as regarding its inflammatory stage, yet by stating concisely a few of the opinions on its mode of treatment, much light may be thrown on the disease itself, and we shall afterwards be better enabled to point out the different stages in which the exhibition of the Bath waters may be applied with advantage.

Sydenham, who had been a martyr to gout thirty-four years when he wrote his treatise on the disorder, thinks that the cure should only be attempted during the intervals of the fit, and that the principal object should be to strengthen the digestive powers. He objects to bleeding, purging, and sweating, but recommends a low diet; he however advises bleeding, if a translation has taken place to the lungs. He says, every paroxysm may as well be denominated a fit of anger as a fit of the gout: in this respect the disease does not appear to be much altered.

Most of the ancients considered gout and rheumatism the same disease; thus Riverius observes, "that a running gout may be a rheumatism, as "well as a fixed rheumatism a gout."

Dr. Cullen advises blood-letting in the earlier stages of gout in plethoric subjects, or local bleeding on the affected parts; the latter remedy is found to be very beneficial where the inflammation and swelling is great, but should not be applied at the commencement of the attack. A little laudanum gently rubbed over the part will sometimes relieve the acute pain. Dr. Cullen is decidedly of opinion that the gout cannot be cured, but he thinks it may be kept off by exercise, and abstinence from animal food and strong drinks.

It appears to be universally acknowledged at the present day, that instead of supporting and throwing out the gout by Madeira and stimulants, as was formerly the practice, every thing should be avoided which increases fever; and that so far from bleeding, purging, and sweating being deleterious, they are often the only means of saving the patient's life. Thus in the regular attacks of gout, the antiphlogistic regimen should be strictly followed, always, however, considering the patient's former habits of life, which may allow some little latitude.

With regard to the atonic stage, the object must be to endeavour to relieve the constitution by producing a fit, for the moment that is effected, the whole host of troublesome symptoms disappear. It is in this stage, when unaccompanied by fever, that the internal use of the Bath water is of infinite service, often producing a regular attack of the gout in the extremities from its specific action on the stomach.

Dr. Falconer, alluding to this state of gout, observes, " the Bath waters are found by experience " to be the best and safest medicine for this pur- " pose yet known; their stimulus on the stomach " being immediate and peculiar, restoring to it " such a degree of tone as enables it to send the " gout into its proper place. On this account the " Bath waters are of the greatest service in erratic "gouty complaints, especially those wherein the "gout attacks the noble parts, from an inertia of "this organ produced by excess in drinking fer-"mented liquors, and exceed in this respect any "medicine hitherto known."

Certain it is that the effect of the Bath waters as a medicine in this erratic or wandering gout is as strongly marked as the action of any medicine can possibly be by its effects; and in the most distressing cases, which have baffled the intentions of medicine, and various means at a distance, the internal exhibition of the waters has appeared to concentrate the whole gouty virus, and fix it in one point. This has been a fact so long acknowledged, that it has been a prevalent opinion that Bath waters may produce gout when there is no predisposition to it in the habit: this, however, is erroneous, as it is recommended in various disorders unconnected with gout, without producing it.

The other species of irregular gout, termed the retrocedent gout, is more immediately dangerous than any of the regular attacks, and requires instantaneous relief. Its management must, however, depend on the seat of the disease; if the stomach, strong stimulants, as hot brandy and water, æther, camphor, volatile alkali, &c.; if the lungs, heart, or head, bleeding to the fullest extent.

Notwithstanding the Bath waters are too slow in their effects to give instant relief to this species of gout, yet the debility and disordered state of the frame consequent on these attacks may be greatly benefited by the waters; and with careful attention to the bowels, and avoiding all incitement to gout, a regular course of the waters may prevent another fit for a very long time.

It is a fact long since acknowledged, that gout is more frequent among the upper than the lower classes of society; which proves very evidently that it must arise more from indulgence in eating and want of exercise, than from intemperance in drinking, as the lower class certainly indulge more in excess of drinking than their superiors. "*Calculus et podagra plures interficiunt divites quam pauperes, plures sapientes quam fatuos.*"

With regard to the proximate cause of gout, Dr. Cullen objects to the opinion of morbific matter being present in the body; he contends that it is an affection of the nerves, and proceeds from the atony and inflammatory re-action of the extreme vessels.

The chronic stage of the gout is that in which the exhibition of the Bath waters is recommended; and never should they be tried until the paroxysm, with all its inflammatory symptoms, has subsided. The great debility, with loss of appetite, and the swelling and tension of the joints, then become proper for the application of the waters; and their successful result must depend on the regularity of their use.

It has been before remarked, that the sooner the patient has recourse to bathing after the secession of the inflammation, the more rapidly will the limbs recover; for if once the chalky concretions are allowed to be deposited, a stiffened or anchylosed joint is invariably the consequence. Bathing, every other day, with regular pumping, according to the strength of the patient, with moderate exercise, will assist in promoting absorption; and were the use of the vapour bath better understood, I am convinced many cases would receive the greatest benefit when foiled in their expectations at the pump.

It has been often found necessary, soon after a fit, to use the bath only for a time, without the pump, as the elbows, knees, ankles, &c. are frequently much swollen, and very tender, and the pump at first is apt to produce inflammation; this is, however, only directly after a fit, not in rigidities of long standing. The endeavour of the patient to exercise the limb, and bring the muscles into play, will materially assist the recovery. Œdema in gouty limbs is very common, but is of little consequence, being merely a symptom of debility arising from want of circulation. Friction with the hand, according to Mr. Grosvenor's plan, is very serviceable; and as the bathing and pumping are generally pursued in the morning, the rubber might be employed with great advantage in the evening.

We shall now allude to the internal use of the waters after the subsidence of regular paroxysms of the gout. This disease, when of long continuance, is always attended with weakness of the stomach and organs of digestion, and eructations, flatulence, and want of appetite; and even after the attacks these symptoms more or less predominate; and so prevalent are they in all stages of the gout, that Sydenham's practice was, by endeavouring to cure the stomach, to prevent the return of the fit.

It is under these circumstances, with great attention in removing the offending matter from both stomach and bowels, that the use of the Bath water is felt with so much advantage. When nausea of the stomach has continued for a considerable time, and only increased by the exhibition of stomachic medicines, the Bath waters have had a most surprising effect; allaying the irritation, appearing grateful to the stomach, promoting saliva, and by degrees improving the appetite.

As the greater number of attacks of gout are brought on by indulgencies and iregularities in living, a determination to abstain from such imprudence is absolutely necessary to let the water perform its cure with any certainty of continuance; for it must be evident, the same cause which originally produced the disordered state of the functions, will bring on an aggravated return, if there be not sufficient fortitude in the patient to withstand temptation. "*Vinum, Venus, otium, et crapula,* "*sunt primi parentes calculorum ac podagræ.*"

We have before observed, that the patient should attend strictly to the antiphlogistic plan; by this remark it is meant, that food of the lightest kind should be taken; not to overload the stomach; and to avoid all fermenting liquors, and every thing which is likely to produce flatulence or acidity. With regard to wine, or a little weak brandy and water, it must entirely depend on the former habits of life of the patient; but the less stimulating food the better. Dr. Baynard was a great enemy to malt liquors in gout, and gives the following anecdote: "I once saw a brew r's dog "that had an *arthritis vaga,* and his limbs terribly "swelled with lapping new ale, and licking the "yeast from their trough and stilling, and after-"wards died of the gout and dropsy; so c-rs-dly "unwholesome are the fæces of malt liquors."

Dr. Summers, whose able pamphlet on paralysis has done him so much credit, in alluding to the gout, observes, "the great number of gouty peo-"ple who come to Bath, and the benefit, under a "proper regulation, they receive, should convince

" us, that the nerves are rather strengthened and " fortified than relaxed by the water ; for if it " brought on such a state, nature would in this " case soon sink under its acquired imbecility."

"The wandering erratic pains are by this means " either fixed in the extremities, or, by gentle per- " spiration, the cause is in some measure carried " off; the vomitings, diarrhœas, and head-aches " are removed by it; and the stiff limbs become " useful, not so much by being relaxed, as the " volatile parts of the water rarifying and atte- " nuating the thickened defluxion which obstructed " the freedom of their motion ; it is thereby pre- " pared, under a due circulation, to be carried off " by its proper secretion. But if this expedient be " long neglected, by frequent returns of the fits " this matter will be greatly accumulated, and at " length hardened into a cretaceous substance not " to be dispersed, and time will but add pain to " weakness, and make the patient but too sensible " of every gouty particle in his frame."

The disorder of the gout is so interwoven with the constitution, that it does not admit of cure; and it is only candid to make the patient aware to what extent any remedy may be of service. None but an impudent egotistical quack ever assures his patient with decisive tone that he will cure him; and whoever trusts to such bold assertions will certainly be disappointed, although he may dislike to acknowledge himself a dupe. The gout and many other disorders may be so far mitigated by a steady use of the waters, as to make life very comfortable; but the return of the disorder is in many instances at the option of the patient.

I have before alluded to the chalky deposits that take place in the joints. In some gouty cases of long continuance they pervade the whole mass to such a degree, that they shew themselves in every part of the body. The greatest martyr to this disease I ever remember was a gentleman of fortune, who resided in Bath many years, and was highly esteemed. This gentleman had an hereditary disposition to gout, and had a fit at college when only nineteen years of age. For many years previous to his death he had lost the use and motion of most of his limbs; the ankles were anchylosed, the knees very much contracted, and the membranes swollen and covered with knobs of chalky matter; the elbows were likewise contracted, and the fingers distorted in all directions. Abscesses were constantly forming in different parts of the body, and frequently discharged half a pint of pus and chalk. For the last few years, however, these abscesses were not so frequent; but in various parts of the body, immediately under the skin, a slight hardness would be perceptible; in a few days it would appear more prominent, and at last the outward skin would give way, and a piece of chalky matter, or, more properly, urate of soda, protrude sufficiently to be taken out with a probe. Many of these pieces I have in my possession, and are nearly the size of a kidney-bean. This was a case too deep rooted to receive much relief from the Bath waters; indeed, latterly he had seldom used them.

Another patient has continually hard concretions forming at the tops of the fingers, (not in the articulations,) and when they become very superficial, he raises the skin with the point of a needle, and squeezes out the chalky matter with very little inconvenience.

Mr. Brodie observes, "the effects of gout on "the joints are very remarkable. The cartilages "are absorbed, the exposed surfaces of bone are "entirely or partially encrusted with white earthy "matter, which I conclude to be urate of soda, "and sometimes they have the appearance of being "formed into grooves, as if they had been worn "from their friction on each other." In many stages of the gout, alkalies, magnesia, &c. have been very much recommended, and certainly with some degree of advantage.

We have been rather deficient in not alluding to Dr. Kinglake's mode of curing gout, and, indeed, all inflammatory local affections, by cold water. Dr. K. considers gout as a common inflammatory disease; that it is not constitutional; that its attacks are never salutary, and, if properly treated, as easily cured as any other inflammatory local affection. Still he does not deny its being hereditary. How it can be hereditary and not constitutional is rather a paradox.

In the inflammatory attacks of gout, Dr. Kinglake advises the application of cold water on the inflamed part, "either by means of wetted cloths, "by gentle showering, or by actual immersion," to be continued until the fire is quite extinguished. Inveterate cases may be combated with ice or snow, suffering it to dissolve on the affected part. To assist this cold affusion, Dr. K. advises glasses of cold water to be drunk continually. He does not consider bleeding or purging necessary; he regards it as a mere local affection, to be cured by local means, and those means cold water.

How far Dr. Kinglake's system may be correct in directing the cure and amelioration of gout, we are not prepared to discuss in this place, as our object is only to point out the beneficial effects of the Bath waters in the chronic stage. Whether his cold plan may or may not be pushed too far is a question; but of this we are well assured, that the Doctor's observations and bold practice, in the management of this untoward disease, have excited a spirit of enquiry which has tended very much to improve its treatment; and that the same fear of bleeding, general and topical, or of lowering the patient, and not sweating him to death by loads of flannel, are principles in the treatment of gout widely different from those pursued in the days of Sydenham.

In this gouty city we certainly do not witness the distorted limbs and miserable cripples so prevalent twenty or thirty years since; not that the disorder itself has diminished, for Dr. Bateman asserts, in a late statement of diseases in the metropolis, that gout has increased; but the truth is, that the treatment of the disease is more rational, and prejudices in the management of it are beginning to subside. Thus we certainly agree with Dr. Kinglake, that whatever measures can be pursued to lessen the duration of the inflammatory attack, the less probability will there be of lameness or distortion of limbs as a consequence; and the greater advantage will be derived from an uniform and steady application of the Bath waters.

In this slight sketch of the gout it may not be amiss to notice the ephemeral reputation which many remedies have acquired in the cure of this malady; we say ephemeral, because we are convinced that, like the celebrated Portland powder, and many other quackeries now gone by, they will have their day, and then sink to rise no more.

Patients, no doubt, have been relieved for the time by taking *Eau Medicinale*, *Colchicum*, and *Wilson's Tincture*, and it has certainly prevented a recurrence of the inflammatory symptoms for some time; but in my experience of their effects, the patients have been constantly troubled with symptoms of atonic gout, neither well nor ill, as they express it. How far these remedies have been ultimately beneficial I will not pretend to say, but the greater number who have used them have gone to their long account in some sudden way or other, and I am strongly inclined to think the *infallible remedies* had no small share in the *cures*. They certainly have the effect of cutting short the disease, but unfortunately they cut short the patient likewise. How far the following case corroborates the above opinion, the candid reader will be able to judge.

B. A. esq; a West-Indian, aged about 55, of full habit and large make, had resided in Bath about four years. He had been occasionally subject to slight attacks of gout, which generally affected the foot, sometimes in one leg and sometimes in the other. His gout was never very distressing, although he was impatient of pain; it usually went through its regular course, and in two or three weeks he was generally pretty well recovered. About the 10th of January, 1819, he felt pain in his right foot, and was aware, from his feelings, that he was going to have one of his gouty attacks; and having been recommended Wilson's Tincture, he was determined, as he expressed himself, not to suffer pain, but to check it at once. I advised him, if he was determined to try the Tincture, to suffer the gout to arrive at a certain height, and then take it, but by no means to check the gout. He took, however, a small quantity several nights following, which appeared to have no sensible effect, excepting that the gout did not advance in its usual way, but made him feel very distressed and uncomfortable. Not finding the relief he expected, and the pain continually coming and going, I advised him to omit the Tincture, and see if the gout would appear and inflame as usual. That night, the 17th, he took no Tincture, and the next morning there was an increase of pain and redness, with every prospect of a regular fit. At night, however, the pain was very violent, and being a most impatient subject, he asserted he would rather suffer death than torture, and immediately took forty drops of the Tincture. This was about ten o'clock at night on the 18th; about three in the morning I was sent for. I found his whole body and extremities cold as marble; the circulation at the wrist or the heart not to be felt; the breathing very little affected; the right limb, which was the seat of the pain, swollen to about twice its natural size, nearly as high as the hip joint, with not the slightest feeling in it. It had very much the appearance of elephantiasis. Sir G. Gibbes was immediately sent for; and in the interim hot brandy and water was given, with hot stupes or fomentations to his limb, but nothing seemed in the slightest degree to restore the circulation. Sir George prescribed stimulants internally, such as æther, Cayenne pepper, bark, wine, spirits, with aloetic injections; but all to no purpose. The whole of this day, the 19th, was employed in using different means to relieve the symptoms, and towards evening Dr. Charles Parry was called in. A continuation of the same plan was pursued the whole of this night, (being the 20th Jan.) as I remained with him during the night. He continued in the same state near the whole of the following day, and expired towards the evening. His bowels had been regularly relieved previous to the 17th, but nothing acted upon them afterwards; the same torpor seemed to pervade the stomach, he took every thing recommended without the smallest nausea, neither had he any feeling of warmth from the most stimulating medicine. He had no sleep; for a few minutes he would appear composed, then start up, and look round, calling for medical assistance, for he appeared very anxious to live. The marble coldness of his whole frame never was alleviated, neither could any pulsation be felt at the wrist. After the first twenty-four hours this poor gentleman was sensible he could not recover; he made his will, signed his name, and his faculties were as clear as at any period of his life. His friends would not suffer the body to be examined, although I urged it very forcibly. I, however, made an incision in the diseased limb, and found it completely anasarcous.

The following case, related by Dr. Sutherland, tends to strengthen our objection to any medicine giving with the intention of stopping or checking the gout. That many remedies may be prescribed to mitigate the pain, and shorten the duration of the fit, there can be no hesitation in acceding to; but let the morbific matter (which it is, neither more nor less) be properly thrown out of the system, before you interfere with its progress.

Mr. Fraigneau, confectioner to the late King, about forty years old. By an hereditary gout, he had for many years been so much a cripple, that he hobbled only by the help of two sticks. Every year he had regular fits; in the intervals he was cheerful, lively, and sensible. Importuned by the great, he took Portland's Powders strictly. He lost his regular salutary fits; his stomach was at last so tanned with a farrago of astringent bitters, that it lost its retentive quality; he threw up every thing, even the bitters themselves. After various regimens in town, he came at last to Bath, where, by drinking the water, his vomiting stopped, but soon returned. By Dr. Nugent's advice and mine he took various anti-emetics, all at last to no purpose. In his case it may be worthy of remark, that when by warm medicines we could obtain inflammation and pain on any joint, his vomiting ceased; but the warmest at last proved ineffectual. With his last breath he cursed the *powders*.

The Hon. Mr. G. an Irish gentleman, between 70 and 80 years of age, had been very much afflicted with gout all his life, indeed it was an hereditary disease; but if not, this gentleman's mode of living would have entailed it on fifty generations. He had been an early martyr to the disease, and had never dieted himself, or abstained from any enjoyment, for the purpose of relieving the complaint; the consequence was, every joint was more or less affected, and his wrists and fingers much distorted. He had entirely lost the use of the lower limbs, and his elbows were much contracted. The principal malady for which he sought the aid of the Bath waters was the distressing state of his stomach. He had constant nausea, most distressing eructations, violent heart-burn, and great dejection of spirits. From inability to take exercise, the bowels were very confined, and the lower limbs œdematous. From the irregularities of this patient, his time of life, and natural irritability of temper, not much was to be expected in the way of cure. He was, however, more conformable than could be expected. After clearing the bowels well, and advising him to take light food, with a moderate quantity of brandy and water after dinner, instead of wine or malt liquor, to go to bed early, and eat no suppers, he began a very small glass of the water. This appearing to sit easy on his stomach, he gradually increased the quantity to two glasses in the middle of the day, but never took more, and after six weeks his stomach was very much improved. For the first two or three weeks he brought up his dinner about half an hour after taking it, and for a considerable time after he felt nausea at that period, although the food did not return. He bathed generally two or three times in the week, and went out daily in a wheel-chair. This gentleman remained in Bath two years, during which time he had several attacks of the gout, but by occasionally drinking the waters and bathing, living regularly, and taking moderate exercise, enjoyed better health than he had done for twenty years before, and the œdema had entirely subsided. He left Bath for Dublin, where he lived several years afterwards.

J. W. esq; a gentleman about 50 years of age, who, being in the profession of the law, had led rather a sedentary life. He was very much troubled with flying gout, and gravelly concretions. He complained of want of appetite, flying pains, low spirits, and a variety of dyspeptic symptoms. After preparing him by proper medicines, he took a small glass at the King's pump, which not disagreeing, he gradually increased the quantity to three half-pints, which improved his appetite, gave him spirits, and in three weeks he had a slight attack of gout in one foot; according to his own observation, it was as much gout as he had ever before experienced. It continued about a week ; after which he resumed the waters and bathed; and left Bath, at the end of seven weeks, perfectly well. For his gravelly complaints he had been accustomed to take pills of *soda* and *uva ursi* with the greatest advantage. This gentleman's amendment was much assisted by horse exercise.

Case, related by Dr. Pierce, of gout combined with dropsy:

Mr. W. aged 50, came to Bath greatly enfeebled by a fit of the gout or rheumatism, (to which he had been for some years subject,) insomuch that he neither stood upright, nor endeavoured to walk, but with pain and great difficulty; his legs and thighs were much swollen, and discoloured with large scorbutical spots. He made a lixiviate water, and that in small quantities; had little or no appetite to meat, but drink he could more than enough. I began with some gentle purgatives, then put him upon drinking the waters, and after convenient time, permitted him to bathe his legs and feet, first in his chamber ; after that, suffered him to go into the more moderate bath, the Queen's, the heat of the King's being apt sometimes, when indiscreetly used, to inflame the blood and heat the bowels, and sometimes to cause a fit of the gout to those that are subject to it, by stirring the humours, and exasperating the blood and nervous juice; but by duly preparing him, and moderately bathing, and interposing the drinking of the waters, he escaped that danger, and his swellings abated, his pains were assuaged, and strength in his legs and feet was in great measure restored, so that in less than two months' time he went back greatly advantaged in all respects; and continued so to be the next time Sir Robert Holmes (his friend) came to the bath, which was (I think) the next year after. I have since heard (by enquiry) that he is still subject to fits of the gout, if yet living.

Rev. Mr. G. aged about 50, a great martyr to the gout, having an hereditary claim to the disease, has been in the habit of visiting Bath every year, about the period when he expects an attack. It usually comes on with flying pains and symptoms of fever, with muddy, high-coloured water; but with very little disorder of the stomach. The seat of the disease is most generally the knee or elbow, and after the violence of the attack subsides, which lasts about three weeks, it slightly attacks the opposite limb, with considerable pain, though but little inflammation. It then disappears, leaving the patient unable to walk (if in the lower limb), and generally very much debilitated. This gentleman has invariably used bathing and drinking the water *immediately* after the secession of the attack; and by great exertion has soon been able to use the limb, though at first with very considerable pain. By these constant endeavours, and the use of the bath, I am convinced he has prevented a thickening and contraction of the membranes, which must have ended in the imperfect use of his limbs; but the principal object in bringing forward this case, which has nothing uncommon in it, is, to state that one season, not being able to visit Bath, he had his gouty fit as usual, but his recovery afterwards was so slow and tedious, and the recurrence of the attack so frequent, as fully to convince him of the essential benefit he derived from the use of the waters. He in consequence determined never to omit his visit to Bath after a fit of the gout, whatever might be the distance.

The late Right Hon. Lord V. was subject to repeated attacks of the gout during the greater part of his life. The fits came on in the usual way, generally attacking the hands and lower limbs. After the subsidence of the inflammatory symptoms, his Lordship invariably came to Bath, where a perseverance in the bathing and drinking soon restored his Lordship's health and limbs. This nobleman was so convinced of the benefit he derived from the waters, that he purchased a house here, to be always ready for his reception immediately after an attack: when he never failed coming to Bath, and always with the most decided success. His Lordship, by never tampering with the gout, lived to a good old age; whilst his noble neighbour, likewise a very gouty subject, and who had constantly recourse to the *Eau Medicinale*, and who in point of years was considerably younger, was one morning (apparently in perfect health) seized with gout or spasms in the stomach, and died immediately.

A naval officer of high rank, early in life was seized with a violent inflammation in the ball of the great toe, whilst in command on the American coast. It was attended with excruciating pain, considerable fever, and total inability to put his foot to the ground. Having some particular service to execute on the following day, which required his personal superintendance, he determined to get rid of his enemy the gout, which it was ascertained to be. He ordered a tub of sea-water in his cabin, and a bottle of brandy, and having first well fortified his stomach, he plunged the inflamed foot into the sea-water. The consequence was, the disappearance of the gout, without the slightest ill effect; and he had no return of the fit for seven years. After that period the gout returned once or twice a year, and went through its regular stages, but without any very aggravating symptoms. Some time afterwards the Admiral settled in Bath, and occasionally used bathing, &c. with the greatest benefit after each attack. In February, 1808, he was attacked with one of his customary fits, but rather more violent than common; and not feeling so patient as usual, he was determined to have recourse to his old remedy, the cold water, into which he plunged his foot, but without the precaution of taking the brandy. The following day the gout had left him; but still he acknowledged afterwards there were many unpleasant feelings. On the next day he was seized with a stroke of palsy, which took away the use of one side, and very much affected his speech. This gentleman lived several years after this attack, but, being of an advanced age, never recovered the use of his side, although his speech was improved; and fortunately his intellect was not at all affected. He afterwards regularly used the bath for his paralysis as well as gout, with some slight amendment.

That this paralysis was occasioned by the recession of the gout can hardly be doubted, as the effect followed the cause so rapidly; how far the brandy might have prevented such a metastasis it is impossible to say; but on looking over Dr. Kinglake's work, it appears he is in the habit of giving his patients, at least many of them, when using the cold affusion, two drams of *Tincture of Guaiacum*, and the same quantity of *Paregoric Elixir*, which together make a tolerably warm dose.

That many of the ancients recommended cold affusion for gout we are well aware. *Ex Serapione de Abynzohar de Podagrâ.* "*Quod* "*si dolor fuerit magnus vehemens, oportet ut* "*misceantur in cerato opium et succus mandra-* "*goræ. Et affusio quidem aquæ frigidæ super* "*locum non est parvi juvamenti.*" But it must be very evident, that a remedy so simple, and withal so efficacious, in one of the most tormenting disorders with which the world is afflicted, would never have been abandoned, and universally condemned by both ancients and moderns, (with very few exceptions,) unless some detrimental effects were discovered. The fact is, there is hardly an author who, on this subject, has not pointed out some fatal case arising from the application of cold water, or exposure to cold.

It will be unnecessary to give any more cases of chronic gout. The origin of the attacks, the duration of the fits, and the inflammatory symptoms attendant upon gout, of course vary in almost every subject; but the rigidity of muscles, stiffness of joints, enlarged bursæ, and the accompanying debility, which constitute that stage which meets the eye of the Bath practitioner for the trial of the waters, is very similar in most patients. To subjects with a disposition to gout, the slightest cause will often produce a fit; thus a strain in the ankle, a blow on the knee, if sufficient to produce inflammation, will most probably terminate in gout; so, likewise, will exposure to cold, or checked perspiration.

But of all the exciting causes, improper food appears to be the most pernicious; and I have observed frequently, that drinking claret or acid wines will with many persons never fail to produce the gout. One patient, whom I have attended for many years, can always foretel a fit by the state of his stomach, and the fætor of the breath; and when he has courage to abstain from high living, and keep up a regular action of the bowels, he can retard the fit for any period; but when he again indulges, gout is sure to be the consequence.

The more we see of gout, the more convinced we must be of the correctness of Sydenham's opinion, that the derangement of the digestive organs is the principal cause of that disease, and that the only cure must be through the medium of the stomach. Thus Cullen, treading in the steps of Sydenham, thinks abstinence will perform a cure, that is, as long as abstinence is persevered in; but he candidly acknowledges, a return to luxurious habits will bring on a return of the malady.

On a review of our short account of the gout; of its causes, whether hereditary or otherwise; of its management under the inflammatory stage; of its thermal treatment under its chronic stage; and lastly, of the cases by which the whole is illustrated; it will be perceived how much the patient, by prudence and perseverance, has this formidable enemy under command, and that the want of success ninety-nine times in a hundred may be traced to the patient, and not to the Doctor. "*Et si* "*quæreretur propter quid raro homines patientes* "*podagras ab illis sanantur, dicatur propter hoc* "*non posse curari, eo quæ natura non valet ma-* "*terias consumere quæ ad pedes fluxerunt prop-* "*ter nimiam distantiam a fonte caloris, &c. ubi* "*natura operari non valet, cum sit agens prima-* "*rium, aliæ medicinæ illic minime possunt. Ex* "*quo patet medicos non esse vituperandos, si* "*podagras factas non removent; et ratio etiam* "*est, quia podagræ nascuntur vitio naturæ, ut* "*superius dictum est, et vitio patientis cum intem-*

"*perate vivant, &c. Sciant etiam podagrici et*
"*si curari perfecte non valeant, propter hoc non*
"*esse desperandum, quia Deus et natura nihil*
"*frustra operantur. Et quod majus est, dicit*
"*Avicena, 22 tertii, Podagram quamcunque esse*
"*causam longitudinis vitæ, intelligendo tamen*
"*debito servato regimine; removentur sæpissime*
"*homines a malis operibus mediante aliqua ægri-*
"*tudine, quibus profecto fuissent occisi. Prolan-*
"*gatur etiam a podagris debito servato regimine*
"*vita propter expulsionem quam facit natura de*
"*malis humoribus remotis a membris principali-*
"*bus, et ad ipsa extrema transmissis.*"*

* Bendinellus de Balneis.

NODOSITY OF THE JOINTS.

THE next disease to be treated of, is what has been so ably described by Dr. Haygarth under the appellation of Nodosity of the Joints; and in giving a description of this untractable disease, I shall chiefly refer to Dr. Haygarth's remarks, and compare them with similar cases which have fallen under my own observation.

This disease cannot be referred decidedly either to gout or rheumatism, though I think it approximates more to the former; and that most of the patients I have seen labouring under this malady could either trace its origin from gouty parents, or were themselves gouty subjects. Celsus gives a definition of the disease as follows: "*In manibus* "*pedibusque articulorum vitia frequentiora lon-* "*gioraque sunt. Quæ in podagricis chiragricisve* "*esse consuerunt, ea raro vel castratos, vel pueros* "*ante feminæ coitum, vel mulieres, nisi quibus* "*menstrua suppressa sunt, tentant.*"

Dr. Haygarth observes, that these nodes are almost peculiar to women, and generally begin about the period when the catamenia naturally ceases. The joints of the fingers are the parts principally affected, but it occasionally attacks all the other joints—never the muscles. "In this "disease the ends of the bones, the periosteum, "capsules, or ligaments which form the joint, "gradually increase. These nodes are not separate "tumours, but feel as if they were an enlargement "of the bones themselves. These diseased joints "generally suffer pain, especially at night, but in "a less degree than might be expected from such "a considerable morbid change. They often feel "sore to the touch. In one case the patient was "attacked with severe spasmodic pains. As the "disease increases, the joint becomes distorted, "and, perhaps, in bad inveterate cases, even dislo-"cated; its motion becomes gradually more in-"jured. In a few patients a crackling noise was "perceived in the joint when in motion, particu-"larly in the neck. The skin seldom or never "appears inflamed."*

This disease will go on increasing till the motion of the joints becomes more and more impeded, and anchylosis eventually takes place; yet, sadly as the disease embitters the comforts of life, it does not appear to shorten its duration.

The observations of Dr. Haygarth coincide exactly with those cases which have occurred in my own practice. Women of a certain time of life, of a low languid circulation, are those most affected; and the disease has gained ground in such

* Haygarth's Clin. Hist. Diseases, 157 et seq.

an insidious way, that many patients have been past cure before the disease was discovered, or rather properly attended to.

In few cases are the waters more beneficial than in this malady, when early directed. The three forms of using the Bath waters are most essentially necessary,—drinking, bathing, and pumping. The first is given with a view of strengthening the stomach and organs of digestion, which are generally very much impaired; the second, to promote a more general circulation and determination to the skin; and the third, as a local application to the tumified joints, in bringing on an increase of action, and promoting absorption.

Dr. Haygarth observes, that in eighteen cases which came under his care, most benefit was derived from the warm bath, and a stream of warm water, with repeated applications of leeches on the diseased joints.

In addition to the above means, the bowels must be carefully and constantly evacuated; for the same torpor exists in the liver which pervades the general system, and which in some degree may be considered the origin of the disease.

If in the early stages of this complaint the above means are properly persevered in, with friction on the part morning and evening, and a constant endeavour to move the joints, success will be the consequence.

I cannot help mentioning two cases, which lately came under my care, of nodosity in the finger joints. The first was a housekeeper, about 50 years of age, who, by some accident, had burst the integument, and a thick cream-like substance oozed from the wound. Having carefully squeezed out the whole of the fluid, I applied a tight adhesive strapping round the joint. In four or five days the wound was healed, and the joint reduced to nearly its usual size. The next finger was likewise much swollen, and being very elastic, I let out the fluid by a lateral incision; it contained the same cream-like substance; the application of the adhesive plaster soon healed it, and this joint was nearly reduced to its former size. Several other fingers were affected, but too advanced to be relieved in the same way.

The other instance was of a similar nature and appearance to the foregoing, excepting that the fluid discharged from three fingers was a transparent glary substance, much resembling the white of an egg—in short, similar to the contents of all bursal swellings. In this case the relief was instantaneous, and no difficulty occurred in healing the part. I have had no opportunity of hearing whether the complaint returned in the above cases, as the patients both left Bath; yet I think it an experiment worth trying in many recent affections, where there is evident fluctuation.

The cases of nodosity seldom meet the eye of the medical practitioner in the state in which the above experiment may be made; but if the local disease could by any means be removed, a general course of the Bath waters would materially assist in counteracting the great languor of circulation, and thereby prevent a return of the malady.

In the year 1817, Mrs. M. a Yorkshire lady, about the age of 53, came to Bath, on account of gouty swellings in her finger joints. This lady, though of gouty parentage, never had a regular fit; but swellings came on gradually after the disappearance of the catamenia. She had suffered for two or three years before she came to Bath, and had repeatedly applied leeches with advantage, by advice of her medical friend in the country. She had very little constitutional ailment, and always paid great attention to her bowels. This lady remained in Bath nearly two months, constantly using the bathing, and pumping intermediately; and where any of the tumours were more swollen and inflamed than usual, she occasionally applied leeches. This patient left Bath considerably relieved; and as she had great strength of mind, and was determined to persevere in friction on the parts, I have no doubt she felt the good effects of her Bath visit.

Mrs. L. a lady of fortune in the neighbourhood of Bath, of very diseased constitution, and irritable habit, about the same age, and under similar circumstances to the case above-mentioned, came to Bath to try the effects of bathing and pumping. This patient was not only afflicted with nodosities of the joints of the fingers, but her knees and elbows were very much contracted from repeated attacks of what was considered rheumatic gout. This was one of those unfortunate cases which was not likely to receive benefit from any remedy, as the sufferer had not sufficient steadiness of mind to persevere in any plan that should be directed. She had consulted various physicians in Bath, from thence went off in a tangent to London, from thence to Mr. Grosvenor at Oxford, and then back again to Bath; trying to purchase health, but making no one exertion on her own part to procure it. At this time she consulted Dr. Crawford, who used every means professional skill could suggest. She tried bathing and pumping, but was soon tired; afterwards, by the Doctor's desire, I applied adhesive strapping round the fingers, but this soon grew troublesome. Added to a very diseased frame, she possessed a great excess of nervous irritability: it was, therefore, not likely the waters should do much good; and such, indeed, was the case; and we have principally brought forward these facts to prove that the best advice can be of no avail, when unassisted by the exertions, both mental and bodily, of the patient. This lady lived for many years a deplorable object, traversing the country in search of some new *Magnus Apollo*, and trying almost every quack medicine which she conceived could in the least bear upon her complaints: but all to no effect.

Sarah H. aged 25, applied to me last winter with enlargements of the finger joints, which were very much swollen, very painful, and elastic; the disease had been coming on near a twelvemonth, during which time she had no appearance of catamenia; and to which cause her medical attendant in the country attributed her complaint. She was wan and pallid in her appearance; had constant nausea, no appetite, and bowels large and tense, with dry tongue, great thirst, and full pulse. Previous to using the waters she was bled, and took some active medicine. The blood was much inflamed, and the lowering purgative plan was continued for a week, when her fever and thirst had very much diminished, and her bowels much softened. It was my intention to have opened the tumours; but I wished to ascertain what sensible effect the return of the catamenia would produce, if we were fortunate enough to bring on a return. She began to drink the water in small quantities, which she increased as it agreed; bathing and pumping were also used, with opening pills, containing a small portion of *pil. hyd.* every night. Under this plan her appetite improved, and she appeared better in health; but for the first six weeks no amendment was visible in the nodosities, and no catamenia. She now left off the waters for a fortnight, and then resumed them, her general health gaining ground. At the end of three months there was a slight appearance of catamenia, and at the next period the appearances were much more natural. From this time the swellings became less painful; she could bear the rubbing better, and they evidently diminished. She left Bath, getting better daily; and if no obstruction again took place, I am convinced she would be perfectly recovered. As this poor girl came to Bath at a great expense and inconvenience, she could not remain longer than was absolutely necessary for her relief.

ON RHEUMATISM.

THE beneficial effects of the Bath waters have never been more fully experienced than in obstinate cases of chronic rheumatism; and the records of our public hospitals, and the evidence of private practice, will prove the assertion, that more benefit is to be derived from bathing and pumping in this long and painful disorder, than from any other remedies hitherto recommended.

As this is a disease which afflicts so large a portion of mankind, and to which the poorer classes are particularly subject, it may be useful to trace, in a concise way, the origin and progress of rheumatic affections, and to point out their division into acute and chronic, for the latter of which only the waters are peculiarly adapted.

ACUTE RHEUMATISM

Is a disease which occurs at all seasons of the year, but most frequently in spring and autumn.

P

It generally arises from exposure to cold immediately after being heated by violent exercise. It proceeds, indeed, from any cause producing a sudden check of perspiration; and among the labouring classes of the community may be often traced to lying down and falling asleep on the damp ground. It commences with every symptom of fever, such as chilliness and shivering, succeeded by heat, thirst, restlessness, &c. These indications are accompanied by violent pains, principally affecting the larger joints, especially the wrists, shoulders, ankles, and knees; frequently shifting its situation, and leaving a redness and swelling on the part affected. This disease when attacking the loins is denominated *Lumbago ;* and when affecting the hip joint, is called *Ischias* or *Sciatica.* There is likewise a species of ophthalmia which derives its origin from rheumatism, and which is ably characterized by Mr. Wardrop.* It may generally be traced to partial exposure, or to any sudden change of temperature.

It is hardly necessary to mention the means used in the cure of acute rheumatism. They are, principally, bleeding and the antiphlogistic regimen; and this treatment is often obliged to be pursued to a considerable extent, before the inflammatory symptoms subside. When the fever has at length been subdued, and the swelling and redness of the

* Med. Chir. Transact. vol. x.

joints have ceased, still a very considerable debility remains, attended with rigidity of the joints and muscles, and great pain on motion, especially upon changes of the weather. The proximate cause of rheumatism Dr. Cullen attributes to spasm, as in inflammation.

The acute rheumatism in general has not been considered a fatal disease, unless combined with other maladies. Yet there have been instances where a sudden metastasis or removal of inflammation from the joints to the heart or lungs has occasioned death. Dr. Davis, in his scientific and elegant little work on Carditis, appears to doubt the fact of carditis arising from such translation ; but from other cases which have occurred in private practice, and the evidence and observation of able practitioners, there is every reason to suppose that such metastasis does sometimes take place.

Whenever, therefore, in acute rheumatism, the pains and inflammation of the joints suddenly disappear, and are succeeded by violent pain about the heart, difficulty of respiration, great anxiety, accompanied by pyrexia, with quick, hard, and irregular pulse, then it must be evident mischief is going on, which can only be relieved by the decisive practice so ably recommended by Dr. Davis;* that is, bleeding pushed to its greatest extent. The same remedy of course is necessary, where the in-

* Davis on Carditis, page 93.

flammation is transferred to any other vital part. Dr. Haygarth mentions the case of a young lady attacked by a rheumatic fever, with pain and swelling of the hands, feet, &c. which suddenly receded on the tenth day of the disease, and was translated to the lungs. This case terminated fatally.

Dr. Kinglake considers rheumatism and gout to be the same disease, and recommends the application of cold water to the affected parts as long as any inflammation continues.

CHRONIC RHEUMATISM

Is, however, the stage of the disease in which the Bath waters are particularly recommended. Cullen defines a purely chronic rheumatism as follows: "When there is no degree of pyrexia (or fever) "remaining, when the pained joints are without "redness, when they are cold and stiff, when they "cannot easily be made to sweat; or when, while "a free and warm sweat is brought out on the rest "of the body, it is only clammy and cold on the "pained joints, and when especially the pains of "these joints are increased by cold, and relieved by "heat, applied to them."

It is, however, certain, that many chronic rheumatic pains are much increased by heat, as the poor patient can often testify when he gets warm in bed.

Yet this observation does not hold good with regard to the warm bath, as instances continually occur, where the patient is immediately relieved, although suffering severely the instant before.

Rheumatic pains will be severely felt after violent injuries, such as fractures, dislocations, contusions, &c.; and in these cases the patient is particularly sensible of every change of weather. Two cases are mentioned, one arising from fracture of the arm, the other from fracture of the knee-pan, in both of which the pains were very distressing, and were cured by a course of the waters.

Rheumatism and gout, though somewhat resembling each other, may be easily distinguished. The swelling of the former, which generally occurs in the larger joints, leaves an apparent thickening of the membranes of the joints, and a rigidity of muscles, very different from the chalky concretions which deposit about the small joints of gouty subjects. The rheumatic patient is also extremely susceptible of every change of weather; and the removal of chronic rheumatism is very much accelerated or retarded by the dry or humid state of the atmosphere.

Bathing and pumping are the remedies particularly recommended in this stage of rheumatism; and the cases related will clearly point out how necessary it is to apply to the Bath waters immediately after the inflammatory symptoms have subsided, if speedy and permanent benefit be expected from their application.

Dr. Haygarth, in his Observations on Rheumatic Fever, bears testimony to the benefit and assistance derived from pumping, and the bath, in cases of stiffened joints. Their effect is to obtain a free circulation through the vessels of the part, and to restore activity and vigour to the debilitated fibres.

Of all diseases, rheumatism and gout are most liable to relapse, and the frequent recurrence of either one or the other produces thickening of the membranes, and adhesions which finally terminate in anchylosis.

Anchylosis, however, more rarely takes place in rheumatism than in gout; the joints become stiff principally from contractions of the tendons, not, as is the case in gout, from disease of the joint. This circumstance shews the necessity of perseverance in the warm bath, which will ultimately relax the tendons of the muscles, though at first they may appear very obstinate. On this account I am inclined to think a much longer stay in the bath may be practised with advantage in this disease than is usually advised. One hour, or even two hours, by gradually increasing the time, have been borne by many invalids, and the benefit appears to increase with the period. Friction is also of the greatest service, and may be used at least half an hour morning and evening.

Dr. Balfour's system of bandaging the affected limbs is in many instances of the greatest service; indeed, in some cases of an inflammatory nature I have tried it with good effect; but it is seldom the patient can be persuaded to persevere long enough in its use, as at first it is apt to aggravate the pain.

The speedy recovery in all cases must not only depend on the early application of the waters, but also on sufficient time being allowed for them to produce their proper effects. The registry of our hospitals, the experience of Drs. Pierce, Oliver, Charlton, Falconer, &c. all prove the powerful assistance of the hot springs in these particular cases; but we must again repeat, that as much exertion as possible is necessary on the part of the patient, by using moderate exercise, to overcome the stiffness of the limbs. That the effort is painful, there can be no doubt; but if the patient give way to his feelings, loss of motion must be the consequence. The great celebrity so justly acquired by Mr. Grosvenor, of Oxford, arose from this grand fundamental principle; and those patients who would not persevere in his plans of *exertion*, of course received no benefit from his advice.

According to Dr. Falconer's statement, there were admitted into the Bath Hospital, from May, 1785, to Nov. 1793, 424 rheumatic cases, of which 386 were cured and relieved, and 38 only no better and dead. Can there be a stronger proof of the beneficial effects of warm bathing? and it is more than probable that most of the above cases were not sent to Bath, until every other means were applied without success.

It is hardly necessary to enter into any further observations respecting the treatment, diet, exercise, &c. in this particular complaint, as every direction recommended under these heads while treating of gout is equally applicable to chronic rheumatism. Although the causes of these two diseases are certainly different, yet their symptoms, their modes of attack, their paroxysms, and their treatment (with some limitations), are almost exactly similar, whether alluding to their inflammatory or to their chronic stages. The same exertions are decidedly necessary, both bodily and mental; and by the patient's own energies will he stand or fall.

A butler to a family in the neighbourhood of Bristol, but at that time resident in Bath, by some imprudence was attacked with a violent rheumatic fever. His elbows, wrists, knees, and ankles, were alternately swelled and inflamed; and the slightest weight or pressure on the affected part caused the most agonizing pain. The fever ran very high, and the chest was very much affected with difficulty of respiration. Every means were used to subdue the inflammatory symptoms, and bleeding was pushed to a considerable extent; indeed, the inflammation of the chest was so alarming, that he was several times obliged to be bled morning and evening. It is hardly necessary to state the whole of this poor fellow's sufferings, or the means which were used to remove them. Suffice to say, after an illness of upwards of four months, and contrary to the expectations of every one, the skeleton of a human being remained with enormous joints. He was as helpless as an infant, and had not strength sufficient in his arms to feed himself. His pulse at this period kept up to 120, and till he gradually recovered his strength, was never reduced; plainly proving, that quickness of pulse in certain stages of disease may arise from debility, and not from inflammation. In about five months from the commencement of the disease he began bathing and pumping. At that time all the inflammatory symptoms had subsided, leaving considerable thickening of the membranes surrounding the joints, and almost total inability of motion. He was obliged to be supported in the bath by the guides, and it was a considerable time before he was able to stand alone. By persevering in bathing and pumping, with the aid of tonic medicines, &c. he was gradually restored; though it was nearly a twelvemonth before he could walk as he had formerly done. It is near five years since the attack, and the patient (whom I see continually) is remarkably stout and well, and never had the slightest return.

Mr. H. P., a gentleman from the West of England, very subject to rheumatic affections, was seized with a violent pain in what he termed the "lock of the "shoulder joint." There was no appearance of inflammation, and his general health was good: the pain extended down the whole of the arm, and occasioned a very unpleasant tingling of the fingers, and the whole limb was so much weakened as to prevent his holding the razor to shave himself, which he had always been accustomed to do. This pain was not constant; in the day he was free from it; but at night, when warm in bed, the pain was very acute. For a considerable time opiates were necessary at night, which, together with pumping and bathing for about six weeks, entirely dissipated all the unpleasant symptoms, and left nothing but weakness in the limb, which time has since removed.

The following six cases are taken from Drs. Charlton and Oliver, being extracted from the public records of the Bath Hospital. The impossibility of any species of collusion from such a source must stamp a double value on the efficacy of the Bath waters; and consequently we always should prefer giving our authority from public documents, rather than from private practice, unless well attested.

James Cole, about 36 years of age, has been grievously afflicted for these five weeks last past with rheumatic pains and tumours, together with great weakness of both legs and thighs, which (though in all other respects he is in good health) renders him entirely incapable of labour, and obliges him to be dependant on his parish for his own and his family's support.

This man, about twelve weeks before his admission into the Hospital, sat down on a moist place, being then heated by working; the next morning he found pains about the *os coccygis,* and upwards through the back bone to the second vertebræ of the loins; thence it descended along the muscles of the left thigh and leg, and soon after through the muscles of the same parts of the right side. The knees were swelled, with a sensation of a dead numbness. He was always easier when he was warm in bed. Three days after this seizure he was bled, but not relieved. He was purged five times, and used an ointment to his knees. From these means he found little or no advantage. After a gentle purge, he began to bathe, and to drink the waters, a pint and a half a day; he soon found his pains relieved, and by continuing in this course, without any medicine, he grew quite well, and was discharged cured in the beginning of November.

Mary Scriggins has for six or seven years past been at intervals afflicted with violent pains in her limbs, which have been generally deemed rheumatic; but within these twelvemonths she has been rendered mostly incapable of her service, and now wholly so. Last autumn she went to Bath for some weeks, and received great advantage by the use of the waters. However, in this time she had spent the little money she had saved in service, so far as to disable her from going to Bath again at her own expense; and as she finds her disorder coming on apace, she is very desirous, if it may be thought well of, to be admitted into the hospital. She is about 40 years of age, of a pretty good constitution naturally, and has few or no complaints to make, except these great pains, and weakness in her limbs, especially her arms and hands.

In consequence of the above she was admitted into the Bath Hospital.

This patient had been regular as to her menses during the whole course of her illness, and continued so while she was in the hospital. Her first complaint was a pain in her hip joint, from whence it was removed by the use of opodeldoc, with which the part was frequently embrocated. The pains then flew about her, and attacked several other joints. At that time the strange infatuation about Glastonbury water overspread the neighbourhood, and she went thither among the crowds of deluded people. She staid there seven weeks, drank half a pint of the water a day, and bathed eleven times; when she had finished this course, her pains were greatly increased, and her joints so much swollen, that her limbs had almost lost all motion. Last autumn she came to Bath, drank these waters, bathed, and found much benefit, as her case declares. She came again, and was admitted into the hospital. When I first saw her, she complained of great pains in all her joints, which were stiff, and could not be moved without much difficulty, especially the vertebræ of the neck. Her ankles were much swollen, and pained her so much, if she endeavoured to stand, that she immediately fell down, if not supported. She was of a good habit of body; the viscera were sound, and performed their duty regularly.

Upon her admission we took nine ounces of blood from her arm; the next day purged her gently; then she began to drink three half-pints of the Bath water a day, and bathed twice a week. By this course her pains gradually abated, the gummy swellings at her joints were dispersed, she could turn her head and neck without uneasiness, and her ankles grew so strong that she could walk almost as well as ever. In this state she was discharged from the hospital, cured, after a treatment of five months.

George Pope, a soldier, about 45 years of age, well made, muscular, and of a sanguine constitution. He supposes that his disease arose from lying on the cold wet ground. About ten years ago he first felt a very sharp pain in his left knee, without any swelling of the part. Three months afterwards the right knee was affected with the same sort of pain, which did not relieve the left knee at all. In this condition he returned to England, a year and a half after his first attack of pain. Soon after he began to feel flying pains all over his body; his joints, vertebræ, and sternum, upon motion or pressure, might be heard or felt to crackle, as is usual in scorbutic habits. His pains were always greatest in hot weather. He was sent to Guy's Hospital a year and a half ago; he staid there twenty weeks, and was discharged incurable. He then returned to his regiment, and was discharged as unfit for service, having lost many motions of his right arm, and being not able to walk without great pain and difficulty.

He was afterwards admitted into our Hospital. After three months I examined him, and found his pains were much ceased; the joint of his right shoulder crackled under pressure, but no other part; he had quite recovered the use of his arm; he could walk stoutly, and without pain. He was discharged fit for his Majesty's service.

William Stephens, about four years ago, after a hard day's labour at his trade, (being a blacksmith,) was seized with a violent pain in his neck and shoulders, which extended also to all his limbs, and confined him wholly to his bed for eight months. Two months after he was sent to this place, where, by bathing and drinking the waters ten weeks, he recovered his health and strength so as to work at his trade for near two years after; and then, by taking great cold, was seized in his loins, with weakness in his knees, so as to hinder him from walking across his chamber; then he came hither again, and in seventeen weeks recovered his strength a second time, so that he has not been able to get his bread by his labour till within these six months past; and now, the third time of his coming, he has been here ten weeks, and in a fair way of recovery, and begs to be admitted into the General Hospital, having been hitherto at Billet's Hospital, where he finds sustenance fall short.

Discharged much better, having been a patient one hundred and eighty days.

I think this is a remarkable instance of the power of Bath waters, in removing the pains which were so often brought on by taking cold upon having been violently heated, even after so many relapses.

Walter Flea has been afflicted with a swelling in both ankles for these three years past, proceeding from cold; but the swelling has been now gone off for about half a year, and left such a great contraction of the tarsus and metatarsus, that he cannot walk but with the greatest difficulty; he is likewise troubled with rheumatic complaints. His age is about 40.

This man was an officer of the Excise. By standing in a cold, damp cellar, to watch a soap-maker, he contracted a rheumatic habit, being afflicted with sharp flying pains in all his limbs. His legs swelled very much, and his ankles and feet were œdematous. The pains were severe by fits, which sometimes lasted for a fortnight, attended with fever; then the pains ceased, leaving the limbs very weak, especially the ankles. He is just now getting out of one of those fits, which has been pretty severe. He is now free from all feverish symptoms.

After proper evacuations he began to drink and bathe. He was very costive, and was obliged to take half a drachm of *Elect. Cariocostinum* every other night. In order to unload his legs, which still swelled, especially towards night, he now and then took a jalap purge.

10th June. His pains are much easier, and his legs and ankles do not swell so much.

11th July. He has no complaint remaining but the weakness of his ankles, which grow stronger by pumping. He was then discharged, very well recovered.

This man's disorder was relieved much the sooner by the warmth of the season, which kept up a constant free perspiration between the bathings, to which cold weather is very unfavourable. When this great evacuation was checked by the autumnal winds, his pains returned, and upon his own petition he was re-admitted.

" May it please the worthy Gentlemen, Doctors, and
" Surgeons, to the General Hospital in Bath, the humble
" petition of Walter Flea humbly sheweth,—that

"whereas Walter Flea, of Calne, in the county of "Wilts, was some time since a patient in the above-"named house, and was turned out cured; but having "since a relapse of my disorder, humbly implore the "worthy gentlemen for a re-admittance, which will in-"finitely oblige

"Your afflicted humble servant,

"WALTER FLEA."

His symptoms were much the same as before; but he did not receive benefit as fast as he did in the warmer months. The waters seemed now to want some assistance; and as he was still costive, he was ordered an opening electuary, with gum guaiacum. By degrees he got rid of all his complaints.

John Beasly, of St. Michael's, Oxford, has for two years past been afflicted with painful swellings in his legs. After taking medicines here to no purpose, he was recommended to the Infirmary at Westminster, and was discharged from thence without being relieved. The Physicians and Surgeons of that Hospital advised his going to Bath, as being the most likely means of serving him.

Admitted 1st May, 1746; discharged 7th July, cured.

This is much to the credit of the Bath Hospital, where the patient received a cure after he had tried all means at Oxford and in the Westminster Infirmary to no purpose. Probably nothing but a gradual solution of the viscid state of his juices by warm bathing could have effected his cure.

The two following cases strongly point out the benefit of the bath and pump in stiffness of the joints and violent rheumatic pains after fractured limbs. In both these cases, independent of great rigidity from long confinement and want of use, the pains in the joints and muscles were very distressing upon any variation of the atmosphere; and various remedies had been tried without effect for the relief of the pain, prior to the use of the bath.

In the autumn of 1819, I was applied to by a Lady, who had fractured her arm upwards of a twelvemonth, yet still the debility in the muscles, and great pain when put in motion, prevented the possibility of lifting the smallest weight; and, indeed, she could not raise her hand to her mouth without assistance. The pain in the injured limb when warm in bed was excessive, and every change of weather had an immediate effect on the fractured bone and the muscles surrounding it. This lady had tried embrocations to the limb, friction, (which she could only bear in a gentle way,) opiates at night, and, indeed, a variety of remedies, with a view of relieving the pain, but with very little effect. Her health beginning to suffer, she was advised to try warm bathing and pumping. She began with the bath twice the first week, afterwards three times, and dry pumping every other day. At first the full force of the pump was obliged to be moderated, as she could not bear either the force or the heat; but in a fortnight no such precaution was necessary, she steadily pursued the above plan for two months, and at the end of that period had very little occasional pain, and could move the arm nearly as well as the other. Very little medical treatment was necessary. Attention to the bowels, and taking care to avoid cold, were the principal directions. This lady I have had the pleasure of seeing frequently since the above period; she has had no return of her pains; and she attributes the whole benefit of her recovery to the pumping alone.

Mrs. S., a Yorkshire lady, had the misfortune to fracture the patella, or knee-pan. It was a considerable time before the union was effected, and there was very great inflammation of the surrounding membranes. It was several months before she could put her foot to the ground, and then found such stiffness and rigidity of the joint, as to preclude the possibility of walking. The pain at all times was very great, but particularly during changes of the weather. For eight or ten months she tried every means to move the knee, but without effect; the endeavour to walk was accompanied by so much pain, that she would rather lose the use of the limb than attempt it. Under these circumstances she came to Bath; her bodily health was good, but the knee appeared much enlarged, and the capsular ligament considerably thickened. In this case bathing and pumping was persevered in for two months, with a flannel roller applied to the knee. From a total inability to rest on the injured limb, this lady was enabled to hobble about the Parades with a stick; and had it been convenient for her to have staid longer, there can be no doubt she would have left Bath quite cured; still the waters have laid the foundation for a perfect cure.

We extract the next two cases from Dr. Pierce, which are sufficient to decide on the peculiar benefit of bathing and pumping in a disease which is not more unlike in the various forms under which it attacks its victims, than the uncertainty of almost any remedy in preventing a repetition of its assaults. Prudence and care in avoiding cold are the surest antidotes to its return.

Mrs. J. Chase, about 25 years of age, was seized about Michaelmas with sharp pains in her joints only, which ran from place to place by quick and sudden removes; sometimes inflaming, sometimes swelling; always severely paining the part it moved into. This illness held great part of the winter, and so much enfeebled her limbs, that she was not able to go, or stand upright; for which lameness of her's she was brought to Bath in the spring following. She had (besides these infirmities in her limbs) several other scorbutic symptoms, such as a spontaneous lassitude, want of appetite and digestion, palpitation of the heart, and sometimes the returns of those arthritick pains, but not altogether so violently or frequently as at the first seizure.

After convenient preparation she was permitted to bathe, and in bathing we were forced to support her with cordials, her spirits being very low, and her strength exhausted; nor could she bear a temperate bath at first more than twice a week, or every other day. But by degrees she grew stronger and stronger, and greatly more at ease; so that in six weeks or two months time she got considerable strength and stomach, and the tumours on her joints began to subside; the palpitation so the heart remitted, and she was (in all particulars) of well recovered, that she, who came hither in a litter, went home on horseback, and continued the autumn and winter following free from a relapse; but came again (whether the next or second summer following I cannot well remember) to confirm what she had got the first season. This lady, at her first coming, drank the waters no otherwise than to quench thirst in the bath, and sometimes to keep soluble; her case then requiring rather cordials, to which being accustomed, the waters were not so agreeable; at the second coming she drank them more freely. She continued after this many years very well, and free from this painful distemper.

Mrs. Martha Greswold, aged 23 years, was brought hither, and was so weak as not to be able to use her hand or foot, nor so much as to lift her hand to her head, but was carried from place to place, and lifted into and out of her bed. Her head also was concerned in this her general weakness; she apprehended every thing that was said to her, but remembered little or nothing. After taking cold, this wandering arthritick pain took first one knee, after awhile the other, and so leaped from joint to joint, till it had gone all over her limbs. She was let blood, purged, fomented, sweated, &c. after which (at eleven weeks end) she came to Bath with no small difficulty.

Her weakness first required cordials, which were ordered for her; afterward I gave her antiscorbutics, chalybeates, cephalicks, &c. with necessary preparatives for drinking the waters and bathing, by which, in little more than a week's time, she had ease, and by degrees got strength also, though under the fatigues of bathing and pumping, and sometimes purging; insomuch, that at seven weeks' end she rode homewards forty miles the first day, and that after ten o'clock. She got home well, and kept free from this distemper.

Many other cases of general rheumatism might be noted, for it is a disease more prevalent than any other complaint with which the humidity of our variable climate afflicts us; but sufficient has been recorded to shew the advantage of warm bathing in restoring that balance of the circulation, the obstruction of which may be justly considered the immediate cause of the disorder.

We shall next consider the varieties of rheumatic affection under the different forms of

LUMBAGO,
SCIATICA, and
TIC DOULOUREUX.

LUMBAGO

Is a rheumatic affection of the muscles about the loins. It is often one of the attendant symptoms of general rheumatism, but it more frequently attacks the patient as a chronic disease, without any accompaniment of inflammatory symptoms. It is distinguished by a violent pain about the region of the loins, which incapacitates the patient from either standing upright, or, when lying in bed, from the slightest motion.

Its causes are similar to other rheumatic affections, but lumbago often arises from sitting on a damp seat, getting wet on horseback, or lying on the damp ground. It likewise sometimes occurs from severe strains, and spasms after violent exertions, and then is wholly confined to the muscles. If attended with any inflammation, that must be subdued; and afterwards the warm bath and pumping will be found of the greatest benefit.

The deep-seated pains arising from lumbar abscess very much resemble lumbago; thus Dr. Oliver, alluding to cases of lumbago not deriving benefit from the Bath waters, has mentioned their terminating in suppuration. The truth appears to be, his cases were decidedly scrophulous affections, which went through their regular progress, and terminated in genuine lumbar abscess, lumbago never ending in suppuration. In the former cases the application of the waters would be prejudicial, in the latter the benefit is most decided.

This disease is very difficult to distinguish sometimes from violent nephritic pains, as the great uneasiness not only extends about the kidnies, but often appears to pass round in the direction of the ureter towards the bladder. It is not, however, attended with sickness.

The principal benefit derived from the waters in this affection is from bathing, and the use of the pump to the amount of three or four hundred strokes, whilst in the bath. The pain about the loins is generally too severe to allow the use of the dry pump, but the stream of water moderated by the bath has a wonderfully agreeable sensation, as I have myself experienced in this troublesome disorder.

If the patient can stay in twenty or even thirty minutes without great fatigue, he will experience more benefit; and after coming out of the bath, the loins should be well rubbed with warm flannel, and he should go home and lie in bed between the blankets. Warm embrocations are also of great service, and indeed friction of any kind. The bathing and pumping may be repeated each day till the pain is removed; and by attention to the bowels, care should be taken to keep down fever. In resuming the usual avocations, the body should be additionally clothed.

Cases of lumbago are so similar in their attacks and mode of treatment, that we shall not specify any particular ones, as they could not throw any additional information on the subject.

ISCHIAS, or SCIATICA.

By the above terms are meant simply—a rheumatic affection of the hip joint, arising from accidental causes, such as exposure to cold, checked perspiration from wet, or wearing damp clothes, &c. It consists in a violent pain of the hip joint, extending along the course of the sciatic nerve. This disease, though sometimes attended with inflammation, is most frequently a chronic complaint.

There is no species of rheumatism more obstinate, or more difficult to relieve, than some cases of sciatica; the most powerful applications, such as cupping, leeches, blisters, &c. together with internal remedies, such as mercury, opium, arsenic, hemlock, and violent purgatives, are frequently administered without the smallest benefit.

It often comes on at regular periods with the most excruciating gnawing pains, and after continuing some hours, leaves the patient gradually, without the smallest pain or inconvenience being felt in the affected part, until the return of the paroxysm. From the obstinacy of this disease, and the mode of its attacks, it appears most probably to arise from an inflammation of the periosteum or membrane immediately covering the bone.

Dr. Charlton states, that in twelve years there were admitted into the hospital 296 hip cases. Of these 192 were perfectly cured, or greatly benefited;

two received no benefit, two died, one was discharged for irregularity, and 99 were improper to be continued.

Dr. Falconer, in a treatise on hip cases, seems to consider this as a distinct disease from either gout, rheumatism, or even psoadic abscess. He gives a statement of the number of hip cases admitted into the Bath Hospital from May, 1785, to April, 1801. The numbers were 556; of which 382 were cured and relieved, 37 no better and dead, 122 improper cases, 13 discharged for irregularity, and 2 died of small-pox. Out of the 122 designated as improper cases, in 97 matter was discovered to have formed; this more strongly marks the benefit of the Bath waters, as they could not possibly be considered rheumatic cases.

From the statement and observations of the learned Doctor, on the disease of the hip joint, or ischias, it appears pretty evident that all those cases which arose from scrophula, or had such tendency, were unsuccessful; the remainder, which, as he observes, arose generally from exposure to cold, lying on damp ground, &c. and where no suppuration took place, received benefit from the waters.

The truth is, both rheumatism and lumbar abscesses may originate from the same exciting cause; but in a constitution with any predisposition to scrophula, a violent state of inflammation about the hip joint might terminate in lumbar abscess; whereas the same exciting cause in a healthy subject would produce real ischias, or sciatica. It is not at all unreasonable to suppose, that any exciting cause producing a high degree of inflammation should terminate in that disease which is most prevalent in the constitution. How often do we find an injury on the knee produce white swelling; this could never be the case, were there not a disposition in the habit to that affection. Thus small-pox is said to produce scrophula; but it is well known small-pox cannot produce another disorder; it merely calls into action that disease which lay dormant in the constitution for want of an exciting cause.

Inflammation of the synovial membranes, which arises from rheumatism, though it occasions an effusion of fluid into the joint in some instances, yet it seldom terminates in the extravasation of coagulable lymph, unless there be a disposition to scrophulous affection, and then caries of the bone, and destruction of the articulating surfaces, are the consequence.

Mr. Brodie has given some excellent cases and remarks on diseases of the hip joint in the 4th, 5th, and 6th vols. of Medic. Chirurg. Transactions. He observes, that it is almost impossible to distinguish disease of the hip joint from rheumatic pain, since it has often no certain seat, but is referred to different parts of the limb by different individuals.

In this disease the use of bathing and the pump appears of much more consequence than drinking the waters, and pumping appears more beneficial than bathing; they should, however, be used in conjunction, and very often great benefit is derived from a tight bandage down the whole course of the sciatic nerve.

The patient should, likewise, persevere in moderate exercise, and not be discouraged, if at first the pain increases. An improvement in walking is always felt more at the conclusion of a little exertion than at the commencement.

The general state of health should likewise be attended to; and where the patient has been very much pulled down by active remedies, bark, in addition to the local means, may be given with great advantage.

On the whole, in the treatment of real sciatica, or rheumatic affection of the hip joint, we may consider it an invariable axiom, that where any thing like suppuration has taken place, or where fluctuation can be discovered, or where the pain is attended with cold chills or rigours, and other symptoms of fever, or of matter forming, in such cases the Bath waters, general or topical, will do injury; but where severe pain is felt about the hip joint and in the course of the sciatic nerve, which pain is aggravated or diminished by change of weather, and is subject to occasional remissions, then the waters, steadily pursued, will prove of most essential benefit.

Miss P. a young lady about 18 years of age, in the year 1816 was affected with excruciating pains about the lumbar region, particularly on the right side, extending down the thigh in the course of the sciatic nerve. This pain came on with violent spasms, and at particular times of the day. It lasted, with very little intermission, nearly a twelvemonth. It was supposed to have arisen from cold, and during the whole period only once or twice was there a very slight appearance of catamenia. The obstinacy of this complaint baffled every means science and ingenuity could devise. Opium, mercury, (amounting to ptyalism,) hemlock, the mineral solution, purgatives, together with local applications, such as blisters, cupping, leeching, mustard poultices, and even strapping the whole thigh with adhesive plaster, were of no avail. After the physician and patient were pretty well tired of each other, she was sent to Bath; and whether the disease was almost exhausted, or whether the whole benefit may be attributed to the waters, certain it is, after three months' bathing and pumping, the pains gradually ceased, and in the course of time the limb, which was very much diminished, recovered its strength. This young lady has not hitherto had a return of the complaint; she has since married, and has two children.

The two following hospital cases are related by Dr. Charlton. Many under the denomination of rheumatism, described both by Dr. C. and

Dr. Pierce, as terminating in abscess, were totally distinct diseases from that membranous inflammation which never terminates in suppuration, and which constitutes that rheumatic affection called *sciatica.* The cases of abscess we have not extracted, as the most of them ended fatally, and only prove the inefficiency of the waters under such circumstances.

John Hughes, of the parish of Wrexham, county of Denbigh, was seized with a violent pain in his right hip, attended with a strong symptomatic fever, and an atrophy of the whole limb, great disproportion of the joints, from whence there is reason to fear a luxation, if the obstruction of the joint gland be not removed, which the warm bath with drinking bids fairest to do. J. P.

This man was bled as soon as he was admitted, then took a purge, drank the waters sparingly, bathed twice a week, then three times, and took an opening electuary, and was discharged cured, after being a patient only 34 days.

William Hopkins, 21 years of age, of the parish of Midsomer-Norton, in the county of Somerset. His pain, he says, lies mostly in his right hip, but that it moves sometimes from thence to his knee, quite down to his ankle; he finds great weakness in those joints, but perceives no swelling. He informed me likewise, that in cold weather his pain increases, and that he imagines his disorder was occasioned by a chill which he took about a year ago. G. F.

He was admitted a patient into the Bath Hospital, and discharged better, after being a patient 120 days.

The next five cases are by Dr. Pierce; and although couched in strange language, are very valuable illustrations of the efficacy of the Bath waters in these local affections.

His Grace the Duke of H. came hither by reason of a pain in his *hip*, which caused him to go very lame, and disturbed his rest at night, and had done so for many months before. Having rested some days after his journey, and due preparation made, he entered the bath, and sometimes drank the waters in the bath only to prevent thirst; when he omitted bathing, in larger quantities, expecting operation by them, which was mostly by urine, but somewhat by stool also. After a week or ten days *bathing*, his Grace was pumped upon the affected hip, beginning with 200 strokes, and rising a hundred at a time to seven or eight hundred or a thousand. This course was held on for a month or five weeks; in which time his Grace found considerable advantage, being much more at ease, and able to walk without much favouring that *leg*. His Grace had afterwards, upon new *colds*, or some other accidents, a minding of this illness again, and was here, I think, twice after, at some years distances, and was at length perfectly recovered.

Colonel M. aged about five or six and forty, came hither for the same distemper, but in much worse circumstances than was my Lord Duke; for his had been of longer continuance, and had much more violent pain;

nor could he move, or suffer himself to be moved, from place to place, without great complaints. After some days rest, and due preparation by bleeding and purging, he also *bathed*, first in the *Queen's* and then in the *King's Bath*; and was, in due time, *pumped* also. In *bathing* he took a *sarsa drink*, and continued thus to do six weeks or two months. After the last *bathing*, to strengthen and comfort the part, there was put on a large plaster of *oxycroceum* and *stiticum paracelsi*, &c. and so returned well recovered.

Sir John C. about 40 years of age, having undergone great fatigues in Scotland, lying in the field in the snow, (which lies long and deep in those northern parts,) and being frequently frozen to the ground, (as he himself related,) might probably be disposed to aches in his *limbs*; but about the 34th year of his age, by lying in a wet bed, was first seized with a *sciatica*, and recovered it again, and held well about three years; when, in a very hard winter, the severe cold weather searching his body, which had been before weakened by the same distemper, he was seized by this last and most tormenting fit, which held him two years. It not only affected both *hips* with violent pains, but hindered the motion of those joints; insomuch, that he could not erect his body, nor go, nor stand upright, though before a straight and proper gentleman, as he afterwards was after his recovery.

About the latter end of the two years which this distemper held him, and after the trial of several means and methods for ease and for recovery in *London*, where he then lived, he at length came to Bath. He was let blood as well as purged, in preparation for his *bathing* and *pumping*, which he followed close for six or eight weeks; at the end of which time he went away, not much advantaged for the present, but after two or three months was well at ease, upright, and straight, as before this illness. So true is it, that the benefit of the *baths* appears not always presently, but sometime after they have been used; and therefore needful it is to allow time for the expectation of it, and not to be too hasty in the trial of other means, but to give nature leave to work after such an assistance. Had this caution been well observed, the *bath* had had more reputation, and *patients* had saved a great deal of expense and trouble.

Sir John continued free from this distemper to his dying day, which was not many years ago of a *dropsie*, and in the sixty-third year of his age.

The Lady Dowager B. was seized with a *lumbago*, or *double sciatica*, insomuch that her Honour not only suffered violent and long-continued pains, but was contracted and drawn together by it, and could neither stand upright, nor extend herself strait in her bed. Her Honour had the advice of the most eminent and learned physicians about town; who all (by joint or separate advice) had held her in several courses of physick from the *spring* to *September*, without much amendment. At length salivation was proposed, which her Ladyship utterly refusing, herself first mentioned coming to *Bath*. But this proposal of her was not approved of by any of the fore-mentioned physicians, and fiercely declared against; insomuch, that when they saw her

Ladyship resolved upon it, they told her plainly it would kill her, and came to take a solemn leave of her, telling her Ladyship that they should never see her more; and since she would go, contrary to the opinions of her physicians, she should blame herself if what they prognosticated should come to pass, but withal sent a basket of medicines, which held near a peck, and of which her Ladyship never took an ounce, and, indeed, not much of any other physick; but her pain being violent, and her lower limbs almost useless, she entered presently upon *bathing* in the *Cross Bath*, and drank sometimes of the *waters*; both of which in a few days' time gave her ease. In the first week she could stand upright in the *bath*, and in a month's time could walk in her chamber, and was at length perfectly recovered. I had the honour to wait upon her Ladyship, to advise about the time and manner of her *bathing* and using the *pump*; by all she had not only ease but strength, and returned home well; passed the *winter* without a relapse; and lived many years after free from that distemper.

Mrs. B., a comely young gentlewoman, newly married, about 20 years of age, by taking *cold* was seized with a pain first in the outside of her *left leg*, afterwards in the *hip* of the same side, and thence round her *back* to the other side, and was violently pained in both; she was contracted, and bowed together, not able to stand or sit upright, or lie straight in bed. She was carried from place to place in arms, and that not without frequent complaints of twinging pains. She had tried all sorts of means to give ease and remove the distemper, by the advice both of physicians and chirurgions, (and

I was told also that salivation was attempted,) but all in vain. She was brought hither in *April*, and staid till the beginning of *July*, in which time she was first let blood, vomited, and purged.

She had so accustomed herself to *anodynes* (for present ease), that she could not quickly be taken off from them, having taken to thirty or forty drops at a time of liquid *laudanum*, and that twice or thrice in twenty-four hours. I at length prevailed with her (though with difficulty) to lessen the doses, and not take them so often; and this was done by degrees. Whether it was by the violence of pain, or the too frequent use of these stupefactive medicines, or any former inclination to *hysteric fits*, it was not very apparent; but she had (every now and then) very severe ones, not much short of *epilectic fits*. She bore moderate *bathing* well enough, and was pumped upon those parts where the pain afflicted her most. This course in a month or two's time gave her so much ease, that she was content to be confined to her *anodyne* medicine but every other or every third night, and could put some stress upon her legs, and lie straight in her bed. Being thus considerably advantaged, and the heat of the year coming on, she returned home, and there not only continued what benefit she had got, but in some measure improved it, and passed the following winter without great relapses, but was (by fits) more or less pained and weakened in her lower *limbs*, and therefore came hither the second time in *May* the next year, and staid seven or eight weeks, in which time she perfected what she had before begun; and not long after (if not whilst she was here) proved with child.

I visited her in London in April in the following year, and found her very well, and mother of a lusty son.

TIC DOULOUREUX.

That particular disease which has of late years engaged the attention of the Faculty, called the *Tic Douloureux*, may be classed as a rheumatic affection of the nerves of the face; and when not arising from a diseased tooth (as is most frequently the case), may be considered a proper subject for the trial of the Bath waters. Like other species of chronic rheumatism it is materially influenced by the changes of the weather, or by the application of cold, and has its regular periodical paroxysms.

One side of the face is the part principally affected; it consists of an acute and lancinating pain, occurring in spasms of about a quarter or half a minute's continuance, extending along the ramification of the nerves. It recurs at indefinite periods, and frequently produces tremulous motion of the lips and muscles of the face. In some distressing cases the muscles of the face have even wasted away from the severity of the attacks.

The obstinacy of some of these affections in resisting every remedy, both external and internal, is well known; and a late most eminent and valued physician tried every means his anxious friends could suggest, without the smallest alleviation. Some cases I have met with thought themselves benefited at first by pumping on the side of the face; but ultimatelv there was little amendment, and the heat appeared rather to aggravate the disease. In many cases the application of cold was of use; and when coming into a warm room the patient has felt the throbbing and pain of the nerve in a violent degree, going into the open air has occasioned an immediate cessation of the pain. This disease is very apt to be affected by changes of the weather, and very frequently recurs in a distressing degree when warm in bed. The only remedy I have seen of service was the *Belladonna;* and this was in the case of an elderly lady who had no teeth, consequently the disease was purely idiopathic. The torture this poor lady endured was distressing in the greatest degree; and though generally occurring in damp weather, the spasms were principally accelerated by an attempt to masticate her food. Dr. Crawford had a very distressing case of *Tic Douloureux* under his care, which, after the trial of almost every remedy, he cured by the exhibition of the *arsenical solution.* He, however, informs me, that he did not find the same benefit on exhibiting it afterwards. Mr. Hutchinson* has recommended strongly the *carbonate of iron* as a very effectual remedy in these

* See Hutchinson on Tic Douloureux.

disorders; and has certainly detailed some strongly marked and violent cases, which were entirely cured by its exhibition in much larger doses than we have been accustomed to see this remedy prescribed; and Dr. Crawford, in an obstinate case, where the *arsenical solution* was of no avail, found the greatest relief from large doses of the *carbonate of iron.*

On the whole, although our expectations are not very sanguine as to the success of pumping in this class of disease, yet as almost every other remedy can as little be depended upon, there can be no objection to a trial of the Bath waters.

I shall here take the liberty of mentioning a case, which, though not illustrative of the benefit of the waters, may point out that local irritation may prove the cause of the malady, notwithstanding we suppose that point to be ascertained by every possible means.

Miss A., the daughter of a banker at Birmingham, came to Bath for the benefit of the waters under most distressing circumstances. She had most violent pain on one side of the face, shooting upwards over one half of the pericranium, and downwards extending to the neck. The pain came on most commonly in the evening, with very violent paroxysms; but frequently she was not free the whole day. Her general health was very much affected; almost constant pain and want of sleep had worn her to a skeleton, and this had continued several years. She had tried various remedies, had several teeth drawn, and had been to Buxton, Harrowgate, Cheltenham, and the sea-side, with the hope of advantage, without any relief. As a last resource she came to Bath.

On examining her mouth, I perceived her teeth were generally very much decayed, and full of scurvy; and as she then complained of intense pain in one tooth, I tried to persuade her to have it removed. This she resisted for a long time, as several had been removed without alleviation of pain, and she was convinced it could not arise from that source. At last, however, she consented; the tooth was removed, and the pain for the present subsided. On the next day, however, the pain returned with more violence than ever; but still it appeared to originate from another place immediately contiguous to a decayed stump. I had more difficulty in persuading her to have this extracted than the other, as the removal of the first had not prevented a return of the pain. With the loss of this stump, however, the pain again ceased; and she began now to suspect it possible all her distressing feelings might originate in the teeth, and promised if the pain returned in another place, she would have no objection to the removal of the teeth. Suffice to say, under similar circumstances she lost seven teeth and stumps; went from Bath perfectly well; and when I received an account of her, four years afterwards, she had never experienced any return of the disorder.

Another case came under my observation, where a young lady suffered so severely from this disorder, that she took a journey to Edinburgh purposely to undergo the operation of a division of the nerve. This operation appeared to relieve her for a short time only, as the disorder returned with redoubled violence. After thus continuing nearly two years, this young lady entered into the married state, and after the birth of her first child never was troubled with a return of the *Tic Douloureux.*

A very violent case of diseased nerve likewise occurred to a lady, an inhabitant of this city, where there appeared no exciting cause, and was attended with excruciating torture. Every means were used, and salivation pushed to a considerable extent, without relief; at length an abscess formed in the *antrum,* and a piece of caries bone exfoliated. This effected the cure, and accounted for all the suffering.

There can be no doubt but this disease is frequently one *sui generis;* but still, in a multiplicity of cases, the cause may often be detected in the teeth; and before proceeding to an operation, or using any violent means, it would be well to examine whether any decayed stump might not produce the irritation of the nerve. Although the *carbonate of iron* appears to be so strongly recommended, and I have no doubt with justice, yet we cannot forget how strongly the *Belladonna* was recommended in the same disease, with some striking cases brought forward in its support.

This state of diseased nerve does not appear to be wholly confined to the face. I have at this moment a patient using the bath and pump with the greatest benefit for a similar disease affecting the thigh.

About twelve months since Mrs. H. felt a degree of uneasiness and numbness down the whole course of one leg, particularly about the knee, which she attributed to cold, having some years ago a rheumatic affection in that limb, which made her very susceptible of cold. The principal uneasiness, however, of which she complained, was a sudden stabbing pain or shooting of the nerve, commencing in the knee, and running along the exterior part of the thigh to the hip joint; this pain was only momentary, but so acute, that it would be impossible (as she expressed) to bear a continuance of it, and was often repeated four or five times. The attack was uncertain, but would sometimes recur twice or thrice in the twenty-four hours; it would come on without any warning, generally whilst walking. After the attack was over there was no pain or swelling, but the temperature of the limb was much cooler than the other. The frequent returns of these spasms, notwithstanding every local means were used for their relief, gradually weakened the limb, and impaired the general health; and this lady is now under a course of the Bath waters, with every prospect of permanent benefit.

PARALYSIS.

THIS is a class of disease which particularly benefits by the exhibition of the Bath waters; and their almost invariable success in paralytic cases has tended more to establish their reputation than in any other disorder. Probably this may arise from the greater number of paralytics which occur; for Dr. Bateman states, that, notwithstanding the diminution of almost every other disease, apoplexy, palsy, sudden death, and gout, are much more frequent, and consumption more prevalent, than ever.

All paralytic affections, whether arising from pressure of the brain, from local injuries, from mineral poisons, or from worms, scrophula, syphilis, &c. receive the greatest relief from the waters; as, however, their causes are different, we shall simplify as much as possible the varieties of this disease, and class them generally under four divisions,

Hemiplegia; or, Paralysis from Pressure on the Brain.

Paraplegia; or, Paralysis from Pressure or Injury of the Spine.

Paralysis Partialis; or, Paralysis affecting particular Muscles.

Colica Pictonum; or, Paralysis from Mineral Impregnations.

Paralysis will often occur from a variety of causes; thus abscesses, or any accidental injury destroying the nerve, will cause a paralysis, either wholly or in part, of those muscles to which the nerve gave sensation. Spasmodic paralysis will sometimes arise from the local irritation of bad teeth affecting the face, tongue, &c. from exposure to cold, and a variety of local causes. Many authors have, in consequence, applied *appropriate hard names* for the different situations of paralytic affections; but it really appears a multiplication of terms without end, and certainly tending to no practical good. Simplicity we consider the basis of *order*, and multiplicity the basis of *confusion*. We shall now proceed to treat of the various species of palsy as illustrative of the benefit of the Bath waters, beginning with

Hemiplegia; or, *Paralysis from Pressure on the Brain.*

This disease consists in a loss of the power of voluntary motion in various parts of the body, but principally affecting the whole of the muscles on one side. It may, indeed, be considered as a partial apoplexy; the one affecting the frame partially, the other producing loss of *all* the powers of sense and motion. They are alike in other respects; arising from the same cause, attacking the same subjects, and cured by the same means. In palsy, the loss of motion is sometimes accompanied with loss or diminution of intellect; but this is not always the case, of course not an essential symptom of palsy. In point of warmth the paralysed limbs are generally below the natural standard.

The ancients knew nothing of paralysis as a distinct disease from apoplexy; they considered it one and the same disorder, although they applied a variation of term to define the nature of the attack, in the same way that lumbago and sciatica illustrate the seat of rheumatic affection.

This disease commonly affects persons advanced in life, usually those who have large heads and short necks, and who indulge in good living, and lead an indolent life; likewise those who have been subject to any periodical discharge of blood, either from hemorhoidal vessels or from the nose, and which discharges have been suppressed ; or from general fulness of habit, and want of attention to the state of the bowels.

Hemiplegia, though it generally comes on suddenly, is often preceded by symptoms of determination of blood to the brain, such as vertigo, bleeding at the nose, throbbing of the temples, drowsiness, false vision, &c. ; and where these symptoms are narrowly watched, by timely bleeding the attack may be diverted.

The immediate cause of this species of palsy is principally compression on some part of the brain, which may be occasioned by local injury, tumours affecting the brain, or from an accumulation of blood distending the vessels to such a degree as to cause compression or extravasation ; also from fluids diffused in different parts of the brain.

The treatment should be of the most active kind, and consists in evacuations of every description, with stimulant applications, such as blisters, sinapisms, &c. Although these remedies very commonly relieve the dangerous symptoms, yet the patient remains in a state of extreme debility, probably bereft of the use of one half of his body, and perhaps more than half of his intellectual powers. It is in this stage, when all inflammation has subsided, that the patient resorts to these healing springs for the recovery of his limbs. " *Paralysis in complexione frigidâ curatur cale-* "*facientibus, et in illû quæ est ex intemperie ob* " *aquæ multæ copiam, utere balneo mullo sicco.*" *Avicenna.*

Paralysis varies so much in its origin, mode of attack, and other peculiarities, that any particular mode of using the waters cannot well be laid down. If the patient has any remains of that fulness of habit which was probably the origin of the disease, the greatest care should be taken to relieve the constitution by bleeding, the bowels by purgatives, and the plethoric diathesis by a light mild diet. Nothing stimulating should on any account be allowed; for what can be more deleterious than continually giving paralytic patients brandy or wine and water, because they are nervous and weak? An overcharged habit will only be more weakened by excess of nourishment; but moderate the stimulating supplies, which the constitution does not require, and you relieve the pressure on the blood vessels, and the due balance of the circulation will be restored to its proper energy.

Many affections of the brain may date their foundation to improper accumulations of the bowels. If too much nourishing diet and too little exercise be taken, the system becomes soon loaded; but if, added to this, the bowels be locked up, a double portion of nutriment is supplied, and that of the most pernicious kind.

If with these disadvantages the patient incautiously pursue the drinking, bathing, or pumping, the most dangerous consequences would arise from the stimulating property of the waters acting upon such inflammable materials. "*Plethora tum sanguinis missione curatur, tum frequenti balneo, tum exercitatione, tum frictione, præterea digerentibus medicamentis, et præter hæc omnia inedia.*" *Hippoc.*

Taking it for granted, however, that all these particulars have been attended to; that the plethora is entirely removed, and the bowels well evacuated; in cases of hemiplegia, we should be inclined to rely on the bathing and pumping more than the internal exhibition of the waters. Where this disease has taken place in very advanced age, and attended with great weakness of stomach, in such cases drinking the water may be of service; but in young subjects, where the disease has generally arisen from every species of indulgence, the strictest regimen should be observed, and the cure attempted by local means only.

The bathing and pumping may be used every other day alternately; but in cases of hemiplegia, pumping on the head should be particularly avoided. In addition, however, to pumping on the diseased limbs, two or three hundred strokes along the course of the vertebræ from the cervical downwards has been attended with manifest advantage, and may be directed three times in the week. In some cases I have seen evident benefit from the application of both galvanism and electricity. Dr. Bardsley strongly recommends galvanism; and Dr. Cooke seems to think electricity serviceable, but recommends it to be used gently, not by shocks. Both these remedies have a decided effect in restoring the nervous energy; but I think the benefit derived from electricity, as far as my experience goes, is from shocks, not from sparks, through the diseased limbs, slight at first, afterwards more sharp, as the patient was able to bear it. There is an instance recorded (I forget where) of a paralysis being entirely cured by a stroke from lightning. I have drawn sparks from paralytic patients for six weeks and two months at a time without the smallest benefit; afterwards a good smart shock has produced instant motion and sensation, and certainly for the time has appeared to assist the circulation of the nervous fluid.

Another necessary point is exercise. It has been a constant observation, that paralytic patients recover the use of their feet much sooner than the hands or arms. Some have supposed it to arise from the attack more severely affecting the upper than the lower extremity, and consequently retarding the improvement of the former. This I do not conceive to be at all the case. The exertion the invalid begins to make is with his feet; all his effort is walking, whilst the afflicted arm hangs dangling by his side, and not till late is it attended to in the way of exercise. It is occasionally pumped, and perhaps rubbed in the bath; but that is not sufficient—it should be exercised with a pulley frequently in the day, and the hand and fingers opened and well rubbed. If the patient were required to walk on his hands as well as his feet, the recovery of both would be uniform.

Friction on the diseased limb, either with the hand or the flesh-brush, or occasionally both, is of great service; indeed, any methods which can be devised to bring the muscles into action, and restore the languid circulation, should be strictly attended to; in addition to the regular use of the pulley two or three times in the day, the exercise or swinging of dumb-bells or weights will be of great assistance.

The paralysed limbs being well fomented night and morning with a strong decoction of mustard and horse-radish has often proved beneficial; and in some stages of the disease a desert spoonful of mustard seed swallowed night and morning in a glass of water has been recommended with very good effect.

It is impossible to state the length of time necessary for a trial of the waters in these diseases.

Many of them are very obstinate, and require the greatest perseverance; and the cure, after all, cannot be expected without an annual visit to the springs. I would, however, never advise a patient to leave Bath just at the time he is beginning to receive benefit. If there be any alteration for the better, such as slight motion of the limb, sense of tingling along the course of the nerves, pain, or indeed any change, then is the time to pursue the means with double ardour; but if this golden opportunity be lost, it may never be regained.

Palsies proceed from obstructions in the nervous system, or the interrupted course of the arterial blood, which by means of the nerves is subservient to muscular motion, for the nerves and arteries have a mutual dependence on each other. Thus Hoffman, Boerhaave, as well as Sydenham, recommended warm bathing as the proper means of restoring health and vigour in this enervated circulation.

Notwithstanding the assertion of Dr. Mead, that bathing was prejudicial in paralysis, and likely to bring on apoplexy, yet the above opinions, together with those of Drs. Willis, Summers, Oliver, Falconer, &c. are in direct opposition to this idea, with the demonstrative proof, that in the General Hospital, where so many patients of the above description have been admitted, no such occurrence ever took place.

We do not mean to assert that the improper use of the waters in cases of hemiplegia might not produce apoplexy. On the contrary, we firmly believe that *drinking the waters* is often very prejudicial; and that the propriety of it is doubtful in ninety-nine cases out of a hundred. *The bathing*, however, does not stimulate in the same degree; for by promoting a more regular circulation, and increasing the warmth of the extremities, it lessens the tendency to fulness of the vessels of the brain; and whatever theories may be sported on the occasion, it is only in this way that we can account for *the fact* of the beneficial influence of the bath in hemiplegiac cases. The heat of the bath, however, used in these cases should never exceed 96°, although in cases of paraplegia the heat may be extended to upwards of 100°, with evident advantage. Although hemiplegia may date its origin from high excitement, yet, as Dr. Falconer justly observes, the paralysis of the part consists in defective nervous energy: Herein lies the difference between cause and effect, and whilst we should use every means to restore the defective circulation, it would be madness not to look to the cause of the disease, and avoid the rock on which the vessel has once foundered. In this discrimination lies the province of the physician. Those who act without advice in such serious affections, must bear the consequences of their folly.

Dr. Sutherland states, that in a period of eighteen years were admitted into the Bath Hospital 751 paralytic patients, out of which number 574 were cured and much better, and 177 dead and no better. Dr. Charlton observes, that in thirteen years, of 1503 paralytics, 813 received benefit, and 240 little or none; and out of the 240, 61 were improper cases, and made no trial of the water. Dr. Falconer states, that out of 730 patients admitted into the Hospital for paralysis in the course of ten years, 497 were benefited, and only 31 died.

Dr. Summers, who expressly wrote on the benefit of bathing in paralytic disorders, makes the following observations. "We have a great variety "of paralytic patients, and upon exactly examining "the books from the first opening the Hospital to the "present time, I find the account to be as follows: "Admitted in nine years, 310. Cured and much "better, 208; no better and dead, 99; remain "in the house, 3. From hence it appears, that "more than two-thirds were either cured or re-"ceived great benefit, and that only twelve died in "the space of nine years. All these patients were "bathed twice a week, and many of them three "times. And what is very remarkable is, that "of those who were cured or discharged much "better, about thirty were more than forty years "old, fifteen of whom were turned of fifty, and "five were sixty and upwards. Now let appear-

" ances have their force, conjecture hesitate, and " reason judge. And when I add, that the gene- " rality of our patients come as incurables from " other hospitals, where there are physicians of the " first character, and consequently where the best " means are used, how strong in favour of bath- " ing (with such obstacles) must be the above " account!"

The preceding cases of course included all paralytics, whether arising from hemiplegia, paraplegia, or from whatever cause; but in the progress of his work, Dr. Summers states that 43 were cases of hemiplegia, of which 31 were cured and relieved, and 12 no better and dead; a convincing proof, that even in this worst state of palsy the Bath waters are very efficacious.

Looking with an impartial eye at this strong body of evidence, which could never have been brought forward in private practice, with what confidence and well-grounded hope will the paralytic patient resort to these springs for relief, if he has but the patience and perseverance to adhere to the mode of treatment chalked out for him!

It is of little consequence how the bathing produces its good effect on paralytic limbs, whether by bracing or relaxing; our only object is to prove that it does good, and that the same good effects cannot be produced on a similar number of patients without the aid of the bath.

We again repeat, that in this stage of palsy, which may be considered a disease of repletion, the most abstemious diet should be observed, avoiding all wine, spirits, or stimulating dishes of every description; ripe fruits and farinaceous food are by far the most proper.

During the use of the waters it may often be necessary to take active medicine, and to lose blood; this, however, must depend on the habit of the patient; but knowing that most cases of hemiplegia have derived their origin from pressure upon the brain, the greatest care should be taken to avoid a recurrence of the attack, to which there is invariably a disposition.

Although we have stated the very considerable relief experienced from the Bath waters in cases of hemiplegia, yet it would not be candid to omit mentioning that this species of palsy is less benefited than the other classes, which arise from a different cause. Still, however, under many discouraging circumstances, the amendment is often very great; and if the patient will cordially and steadily aid the powers of the waters by abstinence in diet, regularity in exercise, attention to the bowels, and avoid hot rooms, he will stand a very fair chance of being well rewarded for his resolution.

We must guard our patients from expecting a complete restoration of the limbs; at the same time it is a pleasing reflection, that many patients labouring under hemiplegia admitted into the Bath Hospital, who had been one, two, or even three years trying common warm-water bathing and other remedies, with very little amendment, were ultimately so far recovered by our hot springs as to to become useful members of society.

The use of the waters, in bathing, pumping, or drinking, need not supersede the trial of any other remedies which may be recommended, provided they do not interfere with the thermal arrangements. All local means, such as blisters, &c. have generally been tried long before patients are sent to Bath; but I certainly have seen some species of stimulants taken with great advantage. A few years since the *rhus toxicodendron* was very much advised, particularly by Dr. Alderson, of Hull; but in the case of a Mr. Grimshawe, who had a paralysis of the tongue, and took, under the direction of the late Dr. Parry, to the amount of 30 grains a day, it produced no sensible effect; and in several other cases I have in vain looked for the tingling sensation which it is said to produce. The *nux vomica* has been latterly recommended; but it is a medicine by no means to be trifled with, and much more active than the former: if in the course of experiments it be proved to assist in restoring the interrupted circulation, it will indeed be a valuable remedy. The *arnica montana* has been also highly extolled by Dr. Collins: its success is, however, very doubtful.

It has been a point of controversy whether in diseases arising from pressure on the brain emetics are deleterious or beneficial: my opinion is decidedly in favour of their use, and the following is a case in point.

In the year 1805, I was sent for early in the morning to see Mr. Bishop, an old patient, about 60 years of age, who was said to be in a fit. It appeared he had been seized with a stroke of apoplexy in the night, or early in the morning, and was not discovered to be unwell till the servant went to call him. He was a large man, of full habit, subject to occasional attacks of the gout; not taking much exercise, but withal very temperate, never having eaten a morsel of animal food in his whole life. I found him in a comatose state, with stertorous breathing, face almost black with suffocation, and totally insensible. I sent directly for Dr. Parry, and in the interim bled him copiously in the arm; finding that this produced no benefit, I bled him in the temporal artery to a large amount, and during this operation Dr. Parry arrived. Seeing the state he was in, and the little relief experienced from either bleeding, the Doctor thought it a bad case, and naturally enquired who he was, for he had never seen him before. On informing him it was Mr. Bishop, he exclaimed, "I hold considerable property on "his life!" Perceiving the bleeding had little effect on the coma, or stertor, he suggested an emetic, if it could be given, composed of 40 grains of *sulphate of zinc*, to be repeated in ten minutes, if it produced no effect. With some difficulty he took both quantities, that is, 80 grains, and in about twenty minutes he vomited most violently, bringing up a quantity of sour contents of the stomach, and from that moment he began to amend. This case was not attended with *hemiplegia*, and by proper means Mr. B. entirely recovered, and lived three or four years afterwards; when one morning he was found dead in his bed from a similar attack.

The frequency with which attacks of apoplexy occur after a full meal is a convincing proof of the immediate connexion subsisting between the stomach and the brain; and the sooner the former is unloaded, by whatever means, the sooner will the obstruction of the circulation be relieved.

Mrs. W., a lady about 40 years of age, resident in the lower part of Somersetshire, who had recently lost an affectionate husband, and had suffered a great deal of mental anxiety, was seized with an attack of hemiplegia, which took away completely the use of one side. She was under the care of Mr. Sully, who with the greatest skill and judgment used every means for her recovery; and as soon as the inflammatory symptoms had subsided, and she was able to travel, accompanied her to Bath. On her arrival, I visited her with Mr. Sully: she had entirely lost the use of one side, not having power to move hand or foot, and with very little sensation. The muscles of the neck were unable to support the weight of the head, which fell in any direction, and was bolstered up to keep it in its situation. The speech was considerably affected, and the bowels moved with the greatest difficulty. All the usual modes of relief had been very ably resorted to before this lady's arrival in Bath, and Mr. Sully had begun the application of the galvanic battery to the affected side. As soon as our patient had recovered from the fatigue of the journey, she commenced the use of the waters in all its forms—beginning with moderate doses and applications, and increasing the means as they appeared to agree. Neither bathing or pumping at first seemed to produce much effect; but the sensations they produced were comfortable, and she was able to support her head with less assistance. The waters internally seemed to be of service, as the stomach was better able to take light food, and the hysteria (which had been very troublesome, and came on upon the slightest cause) had considerably diminished. The galvanism was continued daily, in conjunction with the waters, and after a few weeks began to occasion considerable pain, which I imagined a good sign. After persevering in this plan steadily for six weeks, with the constant assistance of opening medicines, we were agreeably surprised one morning by being informed, that on waking in the middle of the night she could draw up the lame leg in the bed. This was the first improvement; which gradually increased, until at the end of seven or eight months she was able to walk across the room with the aid of a stick, and ultimately to walk, with the assistance of a friend, up and down the Parades. The neck got quite strong, and the speech very much improved. This lady recovered so much as to be able to go to Weymouth in the summer, and return to Bath and resume the bathing and pumping.

The great benefit this lady experienced, and her's was one of the worst cases I ever saw, may be principally attributed to her coming to Bath immediately after the attack; for it never should be forgotten, the longer the delay in the application of a remedy, the more difficult must be the cure. Her great serenity of mind and sweetness of disposition contributed not a little to assist the intention of the other remedies.

The following five cases of hemiplegia, arising from various causes, are extracted from Drs. Oliver and Charlton's records of the Bath Hospital.

Richard Davis, aged 60, was seized with an apoplectic fit, which terminated in an hemiplegia of the left side. The palsied limbs were deprived of all motion, and their sensation was likewise greatly impaired. He continued in this state, receiving no benefit from any medicine he made use of, for many months, when he became a patient in our hospital in *May*. Having been duly prepared, he began with the waters; of which he drank a pint and a half for some days, and then went into the bath twice a week. By these measures he soon perceived an abatement in his disease, and advanced fast in his recovery, till the beginning of *July*, when his progress was stopped, the waters ceasing to make further impression. On this account I ordered him to abstain from them totally for ten days or a fortnight, and during that time to take an electuary, composed of mustard seed and valerian; at the expiration of which time he left off the medicine, it having done him no service, and resumed his course of drinking and bathing, to which was added a strong stimulating liniment to be rubbed on the spine of the back after rising from the bath. He quickly became sensible of the good effects of this course; the operation of which was so powerful and speedy, that he left the house on the 25th of *August*, perfectly free from his complaint.

If the age of this patient, the cause of his disease, and the severity of its symptoms are considered, much credit will be derived to the Bath waters by the cure. The effects of the waters, I am persuaded, were greatly promoted by the season of the year in which they were used.

Mrs. Whitby, aged 23, from a severe pain, which suddenly, and without any assignable cause, affected her whole left side, was in a few hours deprived of its use. The palsied parts lost all sensation; the discharges of both stool and urine were involuntary; she was long deprived of sleep, which opiates could not procure; the most powerful medicines produced no effect; and the limbs were covered with blisters without exciting in them the least feeling. On failure of these measures she tried electricity. The shocks were given first on the neck and shoulder, and then gradually down to the toes. She felt them in a slight degree on the neck and shoulder, but no lower; and particularly the foot, though the strokes were so often repeated as to turn the skin black, still remained insensible to them. She was now sent to Bath, seven months after her seizure, at which time she had neither feeling nor motion of the palsied side. She was, moreover, feverish, nervous, feeble, and emaciated; her nights were restless, her appetite destroyed, her bowels costive, and the catamenia deficient. Much preparation was in this case necessary. As soon as it was thought proper she drank the waters of the Cross Bath in small quantities; which increased her appetite, restored the peristaltic motion of her bowels, and gradually procured her strength enough to enter upon bathing. She had not been many times in the bath, before the catamenia became sufficient; and being thus far advanced in recovery, she was now ordered to have the palsied parts pumped while in the bath. Her dead side, after being a few times pumped, perfectly regained its feeling, and soon after she was able to move with crutches. These benefits increasing as the means were continued, she so far got the better of her disease as to walk the streets with the help only of a common stick. But as this poor woman could not unfortunately be received into the hospital from being unable to procure a parish certificate, which the Act of Parliament requires, her stay here at this time was not so long as it ought to have been, though long enough to become a proof of the virtue of these waters, and to do honour to that private bounty by which she was supported from the beginning of *December*, the time of her coming, to the end of *April*, when she left this place; to which she returned about twelve months after, and was then so happy as to have her palsy entirely removed.

A Young Gentleman, after passing a very intemperate evening, was, on his return home, flung from his horse, and being alone, lay all night in the road. The shock he received by his fall was so great, that many days passed before the assistance of a very eminent physician could restore him to his senses; when it appeared the fall had occasioned an hemiplegia of the left side. He was sent to Bath as soon as he could bear the journey. On his arrival I found his leg and arm without motion or sensation, both his hearing and eye-sight on the paralytic side were extremely imperfect, and his speech so inarticulate as to be scarcely intelligible. By the use of the waters and other necessary measures he regained his hearing, eye-sight, speech, the sensation of the whole side, and the compleat action of his leg; but neither bathing or pumping, with every aid that could assist their powers, had any effect on his arm; it remained always bent at the elbow, with the fingers shut into the palm of the hand, frequently agitated with convulsive catchings, but incapable of voluntary motion. This disappointment suggested to him the trial of electricity; and as the proposal was his own, he underwent it with greater resolution. He used it every day for a considerable time; gently, indeed, at first, but afterwards with a degree of violence I could by no means approve. The operations made the arm sweat profusely, both during the time, and for some hours afterwards, but never in the least contributed to its use.

Ann Lucas, aged 12, was suddenly seized with a convulsion fit, which, after most violent strugglings, took away the use of her left side. A few weeks after the beginning of her complaint, she became a patient in the *Westminster* Infirmary; where, among other remedies, she was put twice into a warm bath, and for a time was the better for it. But her disorder returning, and finding no relief from any measures, she at length petitioned for admission into our charity. The disease was then of two years standing; there was a great diminution in the feeling of the whole side, a wasting of the leg and arm, the almost entire loss of action in both, with an immoveable contraction of the fingers into the palm of the hand. The viscera were greatly obstructed; she was costive, short-breathed, and chlorotic. She was received into the house on the 8th of January; was purged and vomited, and then ordered to drink two small glasses of the water every morning for a fortnight, with a teaspoonful of elixir of aloes in the first glass. The vomit and purge were then repeated; and her viscera being now sufficiently cleansed to venture a larger quantity of water, she increased her dose, and omitted the medicine, which was become unnecessary. About the same time she likewise commenced a course of bathing, and, after a few repetitions of it, had the palsied side pumped while in the bath. Her disease, which was very obstinate, gave way when the warm weather came on. She then found a daily amendment; and by degrees her side recovered its sensation; the arms and legs their natural motions, though not their original strength and size; she regained the perfect use of her fingers, and lost all symptoms of a general state of ill health.

We have in this case another instance of the fitness of warm bathing in palsies, though the effects of the common warm bath were here, as in a preceding case, only temporary. This history likewise affords us a farther proof of the increased efficacy of these waters in the warmer months of the year.

Margaret Bateman, aged 50, had in general been healthy till about six months after the menses had left her, when she suddenly fell into a fit, and remained senseless a considerable time. Upon coming to herself she found her speech was lost, her mouth drawn to one side, and the right leg and arm deprived of motion. She was blooded, though not till four days after the seizure, which was the only thing which was done for her. In April she was sent to our hospital, when she could not stand, or make the least use of her arm, and her speech was scarcely intelligible. She was again blooded, and took several doses of opening medicines, before she was permitted to meddle with the waters. After which preparation she drank them in moderate quantities for some time, and then went into the bath; and on the days she did not make use of it, her limbs were pumped. By the 15th of June she had entirely recovered her speech, her arm was almost well, and she had perfectly regained the power of extending and contracting her fingers; her leg was also much better, and with very little assistance she could walk. From a continuance in this course, without any other help, she mended daily, and on the 11th of July was discharged, greatly recovered.

The two next cases are from Dr. Pierce: we merely give them as a specimen of his peculiarity of style, containing, notwishstanding, a great deal of truth.

Mrs. F., aged 45, was (about a year and a half before she came hither) seized in her bed with a *palsy*, and finding no advantage by what means she used in the country, was at length sent hither. Though she had been prepared by *bleeding*, *purging*, &c. both before and after she came hither, yet upon *bathing* she apparently grew worse, especially in her *speech*, which very much discouraged her in proceeding farther; and, indeed, I was not very importunate with her for her longer stay, lest the great bell should have rung out for her here; for then enquiry would have been made whose patient she was, not what distemper she had; or whether a due method had been used for her recovery. But with the vulgar (who measure all things by the success) the physician that doth not cure shall be sure to have the reputation of killing the patient that dies, be the disease (or the patient) never so much incurable. I returned her back, therefore, to him that sent her hither, with advice to use *antiscorbutics and cephalics; and never since heard any thing of her.*

But where I have met with one example of this uncomfortable sort, I could name you twenty that sped in their errant; amongst which is one long since made public in the *Philosophical Transactions*, No. 169, page 944. It is one that had not only what she came for—a cure of the *palsy*, but also what she did not then think of or hope for; having been twelve years married, and never was with child till after second coming to the *bath*, (when she staid the whole season out, from *March* to *Michaelmas.)* As soon as she returned home to her husband, (at least within a month after,) she conceived with child, and had five strong and lusty children, at a year or a year and a half's distance one from another— four daughters and a son. The mother died of a *consumption*, twenty years after her recovery from the *palsy*.

George Drinkwater, labourer, fell from a high tree, and pitched upon the back of his head. This accident was followed by a paralysis of all his limbs, and involuntary and insensible discharge of his urine, a most obstinate retention of the fæces, a swelled tense belly, frequent convulsions of the abdominal muscles, and excruciating pains in that region. These latter symptoms were somewhat alleviated before he was sent to our Hospital, (which was above a year after the accident,) though with respect to his palsy he was still in a very bad condition. But it soon gave way to the efficacy of these springs ; for he was enabled, after being a patient only forty-six days, to return home greatly relieved.

In this case the different effects occasioned by the fall on the sphincter muscles of the bladder and rectum are very remarkable : the latter being so contracted, that stools were with the utmost difficulty to be procured ; and the former so relaxed, that the urine was continually and insensibly discharged.

Paraplegia; or, *Paralysis from Pressure or Injury of the Spine.*

Paraplegia consists in a loss of motion and of sensation, in a greater or less degree, in the lower extremities. With many authors, however, this disease has a greater latitude, including affections of the upper limbs, or any paralysis arising from pressure or disease of the *medulla* below the cervical vertebræ; for it is well known that paraplegia arising from local injury will be more or less general from the situation of the mischief; and the higher the affection of the spine, the higher will be the loss of nervous influence.

This species of palsy very commonly arises from a diseased state of the spine, originating in scrophula, or *spina bifida;* or from constitutional debility, which occasions the vertebræ to give way and press on the *medulla spinalis.* It is likewise produced by mechanical injuries, such as falls, blows, or gunshot wounds. It will also take place without any assignable cause, particularly in children. It occurs at all ages. Paralysis and numbness of the lower limbs (either in one or both legs) will frequently come on after child-birth, and sometimes even during the latter period of gestation, as if the weight of the gravid uterus pressed upon the nerves, and obstructed their circulation. It will often arise from exposure to cold, or sitting on damp ground; as an instance of this kind of paraplegia, I once attended a most interesting little girl, about four years of age, who entirely lost the use of her lower limbs from the nurse making her sit down on the wet grass. This case will be stated. Frequently this disease will commence with a sense of numbness in the toes, and, gradually creeping up, affect the whole of the lower extremities; this, however, generally occurs in those constitutions which have either been very much shaken by severe naval or military service, or injured by hard living; and where the disease occurs beyond the age of forty, it may generally be traced to one of the above causes.

Several cases of this latter description have come under my care, and they appear to be the only description of paraplegia that is very little benefited by the use of the Bath waters. Their application has never done injury, on the contrary both bathing and pumping were warm and pleasant; but they never did any essential good.

Excepting where this disease is constitutional, the general health does not much suffer; but from long continuance, under any circumstances, a train of dyspeptic symptoms will appear, attended frequently with distressing constipation of the bowels, and in some cases, according to the nature of the attack, with an inability to retain either fæces or urine.

The treatment of paraplegia (and, indeed, of all partial palsies) must be guided by a knowledge of its exciting cause. If from scrophula, (independent of proper remedies to benefit the constitutional debility,) issues and setons are much recommended, together with blisters, sinapisms, and embrocations; the latter remedies are likewise serviceable in every species of palsy. When arising from other causes, warm bathing, galvanism, and electricity have been found of great use, with such internal means as the state of the patient may require.

The above remedies have generally been pushed to the fullest extent in all those cases which either occur in private practice, or which are sent to the Bath Hospital for relief; and it must be a great satisfaction to know, that, in almost all cases of paraplegia, bathing and pumping are of the greatest service. Indeed, in this stage of palsy, and that arising from mineral impregnations, the benefit derived from the Bath waters constitutes one of the grand pillars of their reputation.

It is hardly necessary to add, that air and exercise, by improving the general health, will materially assist in the recovery of the limbs; and attention to diet and the state of the bowels should be a prime consideration. The food should be light and nourishing; and, under the discretion and advice of the medical attendant, in some cases a more generous diet may be allowed.

Dr. Falconer remarks, that out of 19 cases of palsy from external accident, 16 were discharged cured, 2 were no better, and 1 dead. And Dr. Charlton, alluding to paraplegia arising from curvature of the spine, observes, "that it is happy for "such sufferers to be informed that the waters "generally succeed in this kind of palsy. Even "those the most disadvantageously circumstanced "have been some of them cured, and others so "far relieved as to render life comfortable, when "compared with the state of misery they had before "suffered."

The *internal use* of the Bath waters in this stage of palsy is particularly serviceable; it is, however, necessary, that every preparatory caution should be used in opening the bowels, and removing first every inflammatory tendency. The pumping and bathing may then be pursued every day alternately, and not only the limbs which are diseased should be well pumped, but also the spine, which is the most material.

The energies of the patient will also be necessary in this disease; for motion will not drop from the clouds, if the patient do not exert himself to acquire it. He should likewise use every endeavour to walk whilst in the bath; for the buoyancy of the water will prove almost equal to a pair of crutches. His patience will likewise be put to the test; for it would only be deceiving himself to suppose that loss of limbs can be restored without long and assiduous perseverance in the bath and other remedies recommended. Many, many months may pass away before an appearance of amendment takes place; but when once a little progress is made, the advance becomes more rapid.

The bath which the hospital patients use is warmer than either of the other public baths, being upwards of 104°; this I conceive to be a very great advantage in paraplegia, as the want of sensation, coldness, and torpor of the limbs, require a hot bath; and the head seldom being the origin of the disease is not likely to be affected by its warmth.

With regard to the use of friction by the hand and the flesh-brush, together with electricity or galvanism, those are remedies which may be very conveniently employed in aid of the Bath waters, and often with the greatest success. In all paralytic cases, or indeed any affection which arises from impeded circulation, the electric or galvanic fluid is of infinite service.

In cases which require the use of the above means in conjunction with the hot springs, many cavillers will, no doubt, attribute the benefit to any remedy in preference to the waters; but the patient will have little reason to dispute the point, if the union of the whole perfects the cure.

Miss C., aged 4 years, came to Bath, (with her mother,) labouring under complete paraplegia. About a year before the nurse had put her to sit down on the wet grass, and the child had got a thorough chill, and was seized with violent pain about the region of the loins, considerable fever, and the gradual loss of motion in the lower extremities. Various remedies had been used to recover the limbs without success, such as blisters, embrocations, electricity, warm bathing, &c. The limbs always felt cold and clammy, and the sensation, though by no means lost, was very imperfect. She had not the slightest motion of the limbs, neither could she move a toe; but she contrived to crawl about the room with astonishing rapidity, by means of her arms and the abdominal muscles. The spine had been carefully examined prior to her coming to Bath, and nothing like disease could be detected; and her general health was good. This little patient was put on a course of bathing and pumping, and for four months there did not appear the slightest amendment; after that time she could move the great toe of one foot, and by degrees the toes of both feet. The next considerable improvement was the motion of the hip joints, and the use of the muscles in drawing up the thighs, which was a great assistance in crawling. After seven or eight months there was a disposition to move the knees, and the use of the whole of the muscles appeared gradually returning. It not being convenient to continue longer in Bath, she returned to town, and in course of time completely recovered the use of her limbs. The principal difficulty in this case was keeping the bowels in a regular state, which could never be effected without the aid of medicine. The bathing and pumping was not continued during the whole period, but occasionally intermitted for a fortnight, and then resumed. Although there was no disease of the spine in this instance, yet the pumping on the back and loins was the principal agent in the cure, and should always be resorted to in similar cases.

The five Hospital cases next brought forward, are very strong evidence in favour of the waters; they all differ in their origin and modes of attack, although their effects are equally distressing. Without alluding to private practice, an examination of the Hospital records would produce five hundred paraplegiac cases, equally successful.

Simon Field, aged 25, was brought to the hospital the 30th of August, for a palsy of the lower limbs. Upon examination I found him without the least motion or sensation from the middle of the body to the end of the toes. The first symptom of his disease was a pain which, without any apparent cause, suddenly fixed in his back, between his shoulders, and continued with unremitting violence for near six months, when it began gradually to abate; and in proportion as it lessened, a numbness of the lower limbs came on; at length the pain entirely ceased, and immediately those parts were deprived of all feeling and motion. He had now been in this palsied state for a year and a half; had taken many medicines; and had been often blooded and blistered, but to no effect. As soon as he could be prepared he entered on the usual course of the waters, which he continued for three months without the least advantage. His feeling began then to return, and he could, though with extreme difficulty, just move his legs as he sat in the chair. About the end of December he complained of great weakness and dejection of spirits. The strict adherence to the plan first laid down, and which had been continued regularly for near four months, had sweated him too much; I therefore ordered him to leave off drinking the waters, but to go on with bathing, and to take a decoction of bark. In six weeks after this alteration, he was able to walk the ward with crutches; and as his strength and spirits were now greatly recruited, the bark was no longer continued, but the remainder of his cure committed to bathing only. Towards the conclusion of his recovery, he felt violent burning pains in his feet and ankles after rising from the bath; which symptoms at length ceasing, he went out of the house, perfectly recovered, May 6th, the year following.

Ann Graham, aged 31, from taking cold in her lying-in, which checked the discharge of the *lochia*, and from using fomentations to backen the milk, was seized with a fever, which terminated in a palsy of the lower limbs. She was sent to Bath from the hospital at Hyde-Park Corner, where she had been a patient seven months, and had received a good deal of benefit; for at the time of her admission into our hospital, August 23d, she could walk, though with much difficulty, by the help of crutches. But the palsied parts were still greatly numbed, always covered with a cold clammy dew; were relaxed and flabby, and of a livid colour; and the circulation of the blood in the vessels was imperfect and torpid. The action of her bowels was so much impaired, that she was obliged to have recourse continually to opening medicines. The catamenia had ceased for eleven months. As soon as she had recovered from the fatigue of her journey she was purged with the *tinctura sacra*; took the gum and aromatic pills, and drank the waters sparingly.

Sept. 3d. She was again purged, and then ordered to bathe twice a week.

Oct. 5th. Her paralytic affections continuing much the same, except that after bathing she began to feel severe pains in her loins and hips, and her costiveness being still obstinate, the use of an electuary, composed chiefly of gum guaiac. was added to the course of the waters.

Nov. 16th, she could walk without crutches. The menses were returned, her costiveness was abated, the feeling in her limbs was greatly restored, and the cold clammy sweats had left them; but the pains which were first felt at the bathing (and which usually go off in some hours, or by the next day at farthest) continuing without any remission about the lower part of the back and *os sacrum*, the parts affected were covered with a mustard plaster. She wore this plaster for some time; but receiving very little benefit from it, she was ordered to have her back pumped. The pains soon began to give way, and as they decreased, the sensation and motion of her limbs grew more and more perfect, so that by the 9th of May, being greatly recovered, she was dismissed the hospital.

Samuel Manning, aged 22, had been always healthy, till one day having over-heated himself, and getting wet immediately afterwards, he was taken in the evening with so severe a pain in his head and back, that he became speechless, and lost his senses. By bleeding, blisters, and other proper remedies, he was in a few days brought to himself; but the attack left behind a train of nervous spasms, which affected him for a fortnight, and frequently occasioned convulsion fits. When these fits left him, he had, for above a month, periodical returns of a numbness in his legs and thighs, which were preceded by a strange uneasy sensation in the *os sacrum*, and smart pains in the soles of the feet. This numbness, which always began about eight in the evening, and continued till four in the morning, at length ceasing, he was again seized with convulsion fits for four days successively, in which his strugglings were violent, and while they lasted he was deprived of his senses. Two days after these fits had ceased, the same train of nervous spasms returned, with which he had been affected in the beginning of his disorder. Their continuance, indeed, was short, but then they left him totally void of all motion in his lower limbs; for which complaint he was sent to our hospital.

About three weeks after his entrance on a regimen of these waters he fell ill of the small-pox, and was then in so feeble a state that his recovery was scarcely to be expected. He got, however, through that distemper, which was of the fullest distinct sort; but received no benefit as to his palsy in consequence of it. He returned as soon as was proper to the waters, drank them in moderate doses, and used bathing every third morning. This plan he pursued for two months, and obtained by it a considerable abatement in his paralytic complaints; when, by an act of great imprudence, he not only put a stop to his progress, but endangered his life. For, as he was carried to the bath, he was taking with a shivering and pain in his head, yet, notwithstanding these symptoms of a severe cold, he went into the bath, and staid there much too long. On his return, the pain in the head increased to that degree as to render him delirious, and a fever succeeded, which for many days subjected him to the most imminent danger. When the ill effects of this accident were over, a pursuit of his former plan, uninterrupted by any sinister events, effectually restored his limbs to their native strength and activity; and after a residence in the hospital of 127 days, he returned home free from all complaints.

John Waterman, aged 34, by falling from a loaded waggon, had the third and fourth vertebræ of his neck distorted, and in a few hours became paralytic of his lower limbs. His stools and urine at first passed off without his knowledge, and a most violent pain fixed in his stomach, accompanied with an inflation of the whole epigastric region. For some time he was likewise deprived of the use of his arms; but he had regained their action before he was sent to this place. He was admitted Nov. 11th, six months after his accident. The vertebræ were still displaced; he felt severe pains in his neck; his lower limbs were incapable of motion; his belly was distended to a vast size, was sore to the touch, and if struck on sounded like a drum; his bowels were now grown costive; and it was with the utmost difficulty he could part with his urine. Bathing was first used to abate the pain and tension, which were occasioned by the distortion of the vertebræ of the neck; but as it added much to his uneasiness, by increasing the distension of the abdomen, he was at length obliged to desist. Pumping on his neck was, therefore, substituted, by which he found an almost immediate relief; for as the displaced vertebræ slid gradually back again into their natural situation, the perfect use and feeling of his lower limbs returned; and wind in prodigious quantities being discharged from the stomach, the swelling of his belly subsided, and in proportion to its decrease, the action of the bladder and the peristaltic motion of the bowels were restored. This man was discharged much better.

John Lacy, aged 26, was subject for many years, at times, to severe pains in his back, which at length occasioned six of the dorsal vertebræ to slip out of their places. The distortion of these bones was followed by the entire loss of motion in his lower limbs, together with such a defect of sensation in these parts, that unless his flesh was squeezed with a force which in a sound state would have been very painful, he had not the least feeling in it. The diseased limbs were cold to the touch, of a livid hue, always covered with a clammy sweat, and their blood-vessels preternaturally distended. The pains in his back still raged by fits with extreme violence. In this miserable state he had continued for above a twelvemonth, before he sought relief from these springs. When he had bathed a few weeks, his back was pumped, and he was ordered, upon coming out of the bath, to be suspended in a swing as long as he could bear it; the started vertebræ were then anointed with an emollient liniment, and covered with a soap plaster. Such was the plan laid down for his recovery, (for I gave him no medicines internally, except such as were necessary to keep his body open,) and which finally proved successful, though not till he had pursued it near thirteen months. For the first eight months he perceived no other alteration than a gradual abatement of his pain; at the end of this period he could move his toes; it was two months after this before he could walk with crutches; and a continuation of the same measures was requisite for near three months longer to restore the entire feeling and perfect use of his limbs. In this case the vertebræ did not get back again into their places, but the arch they formed grew flatter and broader, by which means the angles that these made with the others that remained in their original situation, became less acute, and thus the pressure was removed from the spinal marrow; in consequence of which, though the patient was relieved from the palsy, yet an unalterable deformity of the spine remained.

" Various are the cases of this kind which come into our Hospital. In general, all such patients have from time to time very severe pains in the neighbourhood of the started vertebræ; and though the lower limbs should be insensible to the touch, at least in a great degree, yet they are subject to violent spasms, which make them suddenly fly out, and extend their muscles so excessively, as to produce the most severe tortures. In some patients there is a total inability of evacuating either the urine or stools without having continual recourse to the catheter and clysters; in others there is a perpetual and involuntary discharge of both."

Cases of paraplegia occurring after delivery frequently take place, and many of a very obstinate nature; and there can be little doubt that the disease arises from some pressure on the nerves, which leaves its distressing effects, notwithstanding the removal of the cause. I have been witness to cases of this kind in various stages, from the total loss of the lower limbs to a numbness of the extremities of the slightest kind. In some subjects the recovery of the limbs has not been complete under a twelvemonth; but in many cases, where only one limb has been affected, the amendment is more rapid. Many patients are sent to Bath for this complaint, who have been trying different remedies without relief; and in no instances have bathing and pumping failed of performing a cure. Obstinate cases will certainly require more perseverance; and the longer the delay in having recourse to the waters, the longer must they be directed to fulfil their intention.

In some cases of the above description a degree of numbness is felt about the lower part of the bowels, or down one or both legs, during the latter stage of pregnancy, and no means are recommended for its relief, fearing they might interfere with the situation of the patient. This is a very erroneous opinion; for whenever a sensation of numbness is felt, and the patient has the opportunity of using the Bath waters, she should never fail to apply to them. It is well known that many ladies use the warm bath to the latest period of pregnancy; it is often recommended as an assistance towards the period of delivery, and if timely used under the circumstances alluded to, may prevent that partial paralysis, the distressing effects of which are so long felt, and so difficult to remove.

PARALYSIS PARTIALIS; or, *Paralysis affecting particular Muscles.*

There are many local paralytic affections which cannot well be classed either under the head of *Hemiplegia* or *Paraplegia*. Of such may be considered partial paralysis, or want of sensation of the nerves supplying the organs of hearing, seeing, smelling, tasting, or feeling; likewise loss of power in different muscles from local injuries, exposure to cold, irritation of worms, &c. That particular affection arising from mineral poisons we do not include, as it will be considered under the head of *Colica Pictonum.*

The varieties of situations which may be paralyzed, or which may be partially deprived of sensation, and the anomalous cases which continually occur, can hardly be enumerated. There is, however, one satisfaction—the knowledge that all cases attended with loss of sensation, or loss of motion, not immediately deriving their origin from the brain, are much easier cured by the assistance of the Bath waters, and by no means attended with the same degree of danger.

Thus we should class all paralytic affections under the term of partial palsy, which do not come under the class of hemiplegia, or palsy of one side complete; under the class of paraplegia, or palsy of the lower extremities complete; or arising from mineral poisons.

It will be quite unnecessary to repeat the mode of application of the Bath waters in these various affections; the same directions are applicable as given under the heads of hemiplegia or paraplegia, and the same attention to diet and other particulars should be strongly enforced.

It is, however, right to observe, that many cases of paralytic affection under this head derive their origin from the state of the stomach and the bilious secretions; and whilst we are pursuing a course of the waters for a removal of the obstructed circulation, the greatest attention is necessary, not only to keep the bowels regular, but to quicken the torpor of the liver, and relieve it of that load of vitiated bile, which often deranges the whole machine. This cause was so well known to the ancients, that some species of palsy they denominated bilious palsies, and very properly attempted the cure through the medium of the *primæ viæ*.

The cases of partial palsy, which are principally benefited by the Bath waters are those where the muscles are affected: and in these cases they are decidedly superior to every other remedy. Where the organs of hearing, seeing, tasting, or smelling become the subjects of paralysis, little can be done under a course of the waters; and to recommend them in these maladies is only doing the waters an injury, and prejudicing patients against their use in those complaints wherein they may be exhibited with advantage.

The use of galvanism and electricity is of the greatest benefit; and, particularly in this species of palsy, may be considered very powerful auxiliaries.

We shall now state some of the various cases which have occurred, either in the public hospitals or private practice; nevertheless, if we were to bring forward all which come under the eye of the medical practitioner in this city of invalids, a thick quarto would hardly be sufficient to contain them.

The two following cases are taken from Dr. Guidot; the one of a palsy of the muscles of the tongue, the other of the muscles of the throat. In these situations, generally, there is very little benefit derived from the Bath waters; and on that account we are glad to bring forward any cases where a chance of success may justify their use.

A Bristol lady, Mrs. Tapscot, who had a paralysis of the nerves of the tongue, received not the smallest benefit from the waters. She had not any hesitation in her speech, or any affection which could be detected, excepting a total loss of taste and a want of secretion of the salivary glands; and during conversation she was always obliged to have a tumbler of water on the table to moisten her mouth every two or three minutes, to prevent its cleaving to the roof. I do not recollect all the circumstances of this case; but I know she was attempted to be salivated previous to coming to Bath, which produced great soreness of the mouth, but no action on the salivary glands. In another case, of a Liverpool gentleman, where the organs of speech were affected, the waters were of no service, although there was no paralysis of any other part. The two cases as related by Dr. Guidot are as follow.

Edward Shepherd Joyner, troubled from his childhood with a palsy of the tongue, that he could neither speak plain or swallow well. Swimming in the bath, and diving for farthings, as boys used to do, applying his mouth to a cock then continually running, and taking the water to the root of the tongue for a long time, at length recovered the use of his voice, and the strength of the muscles of the tongue subservient to the same.

Madam Phillips, of London, in a palsy or relaxation of the muscles of the throat, which rendered swallowing any thing very difficult, by bathing and drinking the waters at the King's Bath, received great benefit. Before she left Bath she could eat and drink much better than when she came.

Mr. G. came to Bath for the benefit of the waters in a case of partial paralysis of the arm. In the battle of Waterloo a ball passed through the muscles of the arm, without injuring the bone, but it was supposed had divided the nerve. In course of time the wound healed, but left a numbness of the muscles and weakness of the limb, which almost deprived him of its use: there was no deficiency of warmth, but merely of sensation. Previous to coming to Bath he had used electricity, blisters, and stimulating embrocations, without effect. This gentleman went through a course of bathing and pumping, together with electricity, for a considerable time, without much apparent benefit.

By perseverance, however, the motion and sensation were both restored, and he left Bath perfectly well.

Miss J., aged 18, a tall, elegant figure, enjoying pretty good health in general, but latterly subject to violent head-aches and obstructed catamenia. These affections were relieved by proper remedies, and the patient went to the sea-side for change of air. After being absent from Bath a few weeks, she was suddenly seized with a paralysis of the muscles of the right side of the face. The muscles were greatly distorted, and the tongue completely drawn to one side of the mouth; in short, her whole appearance was very distressing. There was no difference of warmth in the two cheeks, but the sensation was dull and obtuse. This lady being absent from her friends, immediately came to Bath. She complained of great pain in her head, and was extremely low and hysterical regarding her complaint; but in no other respect was she indisposed, and there was not the slightest affection of the upper or lower extremity. The bowels were very confined, and at all times relieved with the greatest difficulty. Her sister, who was with her in the country, imagined the seizure to arise from exposure to cold and damp, by sitting in a window with the right side of the face exposed. Bleeding, a blister to the neck, and active opening medicine, were the means at first employed to relieve the head, After this was accomplished, as there was very little fever, she commenced bathing, which, with the constant action of opening and sometimes mercurial medicines, gradually recovered the paralysed muscles in about two months, and the proper sensaion was restored at the same time.

The foregoing case is very interesting; and the recovery much more rapid than I had the slightest conception of, from the first view of the patient. A case related by Dr. Percival, in the Medico-Chirurgico Transactions, is in many respects very similar. The cause of the paralysis was in both from partial exposure, and the age and state of the patients nearly the same; but in the Doctor's case, the symptoms of hysteria were much more distressing, and the duration of the disease much longer. I, however, attribute the quick termination of my patient's case to the early use of the bath; and suspect the other case would have been less distressing, had the same fortunate means been within reach.

The next four cases are from the Hospital reports, and are sufficient to attest, that in this species of palsy no remedy in point of efficacy can supersede the use of the bath. Should, however, the affection arise from the local irritation of worms, it must be evident that no permanent benefit can be derived without a removal of the cause; so in the cases of local injuries, local means will be necessary, before the patient can with propriety be recommended to the bath. But when the cause has been removed, and the general and local inflammation subdued, and the partial paralysis as a consequence remains, then the benefit of bathing and pumping on the spine and on the affected part will become apparent.

Anne West, aged 24, was recommended to this charity for a pain in her right hand and arm. She had been ill of a fever, which, after six weeks continuance, terminated in a critical deposit of the febrile matter in these parts; for immediately as the symptoms of the fever declined, she felt an acute pain between her fore finger and thumb, from whence, in a few hours, it extended to the wrist, and in about a week reached as high as the elbow. Such was the case when she petitioned for admission into our Hospital; but before a vacancy happened, her disease was changed. The pain had entirely left her, and in its place a *dead palsy* possessed the arm and hand, which absolutely destroyed all sensation and motion from the elbow to the ends of the fingers. As the patient was in all other respects well, and the disease appeared to be merely a local one, it was thought unnecessary to have recourse to any other measure than that of pumping the dead limb; by which both its feeling and action were in 131 days perfectly regained.

This case is an exception to the general rule, before mentioned, of pumping the spine of the back as well as the palsied limb, though it seldom happens that both are necessary.

Hannah Loscomb, of a florid complexion, strong and healthy, about 40 years of age, by sitting in the open air after being much heated, was seized with a fever, attended with excessive pain in her hips, thighs, legs, and feet. By the use of sudorifics the pain abated in the left leg and thigh, but became more violently fixed in the other side. The whole right limb began then to swell, and increased to a prodigious size, without the skin being discoloured, or the pain abated; in which state it continued for near a month, when, upon the pains growing less, and the swelling subsiding, the parts affected became more and more numbed, and finally were dispossessed of all feeling and motion. She passed many months in this helpless condition; and such was her state, when received into our hospital. Having first taken such medicines as were necessary to prepare her for the use of the waters, she drank them daily, bathed thrice a week, had the limbs pumped while in the bath, and used the dry pump the days she did not bathe. When warm immersion had been five or six times repeated, she complained of a return of pain in the palsied parts, which was particularly severe after every bathing. But as the pain was judged to be an indication of returning health, she was ordered to persist. At the expiration of about six weeks the deadness of her leg and thigh was removed, and she then felt no more pain from the bath; but by persevering in its use, together with the assistance of pumping, she had the strength and motion of the diseased limbs entirely restored.

John Westlake, aged 38, attributed to his lying on damp straw a stiffness in his knees, which rendered him incapable of walking. This complaint increasing at length occasioned a paralytic affection of the lower limbs, and extending itself to the arms and hands, it deprived all those parts of their sense and feeling, though it left them, in some degree, possessed of their powers of motion. The parts more immediately affected in this manner were the hands and feet; which, notwithstanding their being absolutely dead to the touch, he could move readily enough, though their actions were awkward, and too weak to be of much assistance to him. He followed the customary practice of the hospital, as to bathing and drinking, for five months; and was *minuted* on our register, on his discharge, *much better.*

I have-inserted this man's case, as it is the only one I ever knew of that species of palsy, in which the diseased parts retain their *motion* after being deprived of their sensation. Though as an instance of this uncommon affection, it was far from being so completely satisfactory as the facts mentioned in the Memoirs of the Royal Academy for the year 1743.

Margaret Hobbs, 31 years of age, had possessed a good state of health till within a twelvemonth before she was recommended to this charity, when she was taken with violent pains in the region of the stomach, continual vomitings, and an obstinate costiveness. The vomitings and costiveness being with much difficulty removed, the pains left her stomach, and settled in her lower limbs, of whose use she was deprived for two months. They then shifted to her shoulders, and the lower limbs regained their functions. From the shoulders the pain soon descended to the wrists, and her hands were rendered paralytic. Her fingers were so strongly contracted, she could not move them; and large hard swellings rose on the backs of her hands. Her bowels were costive, and catamenia obstructed.

On account of these two last symptoms, the use of an opening electuary, and the occasional assistance of deobstruent medicines, became necessary, with the customary regimen of the waters; by which all her complaints were cured, except the tumors on the backs of her hands. These, not giving way to the pump, were removed by the application of blisters, and her recovery was perfected in 151 days.

"Pumping will generally dissolve, and by the "perspiration it occasions in the part, discharge "these swellings; but sometimes it will only soften "them; in which case we find it necessary to cover "the tumours with blisters, or plasters, or cata-"plasms made of mustard seed."

This was a case supposed to originate from bilious colic; I have no doubt an improper secretion of bile accompanied the attack; but from the symptoms, and particularly the swellings on the back of the hands, I am very much inclined to suspect, if the origin had been minutely traced, it would have been found to proceed from some mineral impregnation.

Colica Pictonum; or, *Paralysis from Mineral Impregnations.*

This disease, under the appellation of the lead colic, the Devonshire colic, the West-India colic, and the colic of Poitou, has long engaged the attention of medical men; and it appears to be now almost universally acknowledged to arise from some impregnation of lead. Sir George Baker, in the first volume of the Medical Transactions, has given the history of this disease from the earliest period; and he satisfactorily proves it to have been known and commented on by very old authors, but frequently without a suspicion of its cause.

Dr. Warren observes, that "the colica pictonum, "from whatever cause it proceeds, begins with a "sensation of weight or pain at the pit of the "stomach, attended with loss of appetite, yellow-"ness in the countenance, a slight degree of "sickness, and costiveness. The pain gradually "increases, and soon becomes violent and continual; "the sickness advances nearly in the same propor-"tion, and by the second day of the disease retch-"ings are succeeded by frequent vomitings of very "acrid slime and porraceous bile." The pain comes on by fits, most commonly seated at the pit of the stomach, frequently descending to the region of the navel, and from thence darting to the back and loins, and in the course of the ureter to the bladder. All these symptoms gradually increase, with a spasmodic constriction of the abdominal muscles, as well as the intestines, which appear drawn in towards the back. As the disease advances, violent pains are felt in different parts of the body, which at length terminate in palsy.

This species of paralysis principally attacks the hands and wrists, more rarely the feet, and seldom or never deranges the intellect. A wasting of the muscles of the shoulder and hand is one of the most prominent features.

Its causes are chiefly mineral impregnations, viz. quicksilver, arsenic, or lead; the latter is by far the most prevailing cause, and the former, Sir George Baker conceives, only to be productive of this disease from its adulteration with lead.

All miners, manufacturers, and artisans who work in lead, particularly painters, are very subject to this disorder. It was formerly supposed that this disease originated in Devonshire, from the acidity of the apples, or the cider, which is the common drink of the country; also in Poitou, from the sourness of the wines. Without doubt this is the cause of the disease, but in a different sense from what these authors supposed; for it is the acid principle acting upon the lead used either in the machinery or the glazing of the vessels, which impregnates the liquor. As for the acid itself producing colic, it certainly will in many subjects; but the paralysis afterwards demonstrates the noxious ingredient. Lemon juice has even been directed in this disorder ; and it is frequently given to seamen in the quantity of half a pint or more a day without the slightest injury.

Taking cold, or general debility arising from rheumatic affection, or protracted disease of any kind, may predispose the patient, or rather make him more susceptible of the impregnations of lead. Sometimes these cases of colic have been mistaken for gout, rheumatism, gravel, &c.

The principal remedies recommended in the cure of this complaint are warm bathing, friction, electricity, with blisters, and stimulant applications, also by tonic medicines, and occasional purgatives. The use of mercury, even to salivation, has been also advised ; but I have never seen it of service. As a medicine taken occasionally for the purpose of clearing the bowels, and stimulating the action of the liver, which is always torpid in this disease, it is of the most essential benefit. The effect of lead on the system is always to obstruct the biliary secretions ; and the clay-coloured appearance of the motions, with the high-coloured water, and cadaverous countenance, are sufficient evidence how much this organ is concerned in the disease.

Bleeding is not in general advised in these attacks, unless attended with fever, which is seldom the case. Vomiting has been much recommended; but Dr. Warren thinks, though it appears to give temporary relief, that it does not tend to remove the cause, but rather to aggravate the disorder.

Galvanism or electricity do not appear to benefit this disease so much as most other species of palsy. As, however, we have just remarked, that the bile is very much obstructed, and sometimes very difficult to be stimulated, the action of the galvanic fluid passing through the liver has been found to produce an increase of energy, and has brought off an amazing quantity of vitiated bile. In this way it has proved of the greatest service.

It has been observed in Devonshire, that many incipient cases of colic were cured by a fortunate spontaneous diarrhæa; and this effort of nature points out that our medical means should be particularly directed to the action of the bowels, which, from the degree of spasmodic constriction, is often a difficult point to be attained.

It is very seldom we have an opportunity of seeing this complaint in its earliest stages; generally the colic pains, nausea, and other disagreeable feelings, have subsided, and nothing but the paralysis remains; indeed, it is very much the character of this disease to lose all those unpleasant symptoms as soon as the limbs become affected.

All we have to do in this stage is to restore the limbs, and bring about a healthy action of the liver.

Of all remedies recommended in the cure of this class of diseases, the Bath waters bear the most unequivocal testimony, and have been celebrated from the earliest observation of this complaint. Dr. Andrew, physician to the Devon and Exeter Hospital, in a letter to Sir George Baker, states the number of patients labouring under this disorder at 285, admitted in four years. He adds, "I have known this complaint cured radically; "though I confess a return often happens. When "the disease proves obstinate, we always endea- "vour to get our patients into the Hospital at "Bath; the Bath waters, though not a specific, "being esteemed by us the most effectual remedy, "both externally and internally used." It appears, likewise, that 80 patients with the Devonshire colic were admitted into the Bath Hospital in the course of one year, of whom 40 were cured, and 36 greatly relieved, *and these some of the worst cases sent from the Exeter Hospital, because they could not be cured.* Can stronger evidence be brought forward?

What says Dr. Warren? "When these means "have failed to remove the costiveness, I have "known the Bath waters singularly serviceable; "and even when the bowels have not particularly "wanted their assistance, they seem to recruit the

" debilitated patient sooner than any other means." Dr. Cooke observes, " for the cure of paralysis " from lead, and other noxious mineral substances, " the Bath waters are celebrated, and also those of " Bareges and Aix-la-Chapelle. Very beneficial " effects are said to have followed the external " application and internal use of sulphureous waters " in the cases of a number of painters, who, having " been employed in the arsenals of the port of " Ferrol, became affected with the *colica pictonum*, " attended with paralytic affections of the hands " and arms." Dr. Báynard says, " I have visited " Bath for thirty-six years, and have seen wonder- " ful and most deplorable cases there cured, and " some in a very little time, (where care and cau- " tion have been observed,) especially in the West- " India gripes and colics, where a paralysis has " been general; and others with arms, hands, and " legs, strangely contracted."

The regimen proper for patients labouring under this disease may be more generous than what is at all advisable under any other class of palsy. The food should be light and easy of digestion, and withal nourishing; but wine, spirits, or stimulating food are highly improper.

Notwithstanding many of the upper classes in society, from accidental exposure to the impregnation of mineral substances, become the victims of this formidable disease, yet by far the greatest portion are poor mechanics, labourers, or painters, who, if they fail of recovery, have no other prospect than a workhouse to end their miserable days. But if, through the slightness of the attack, or the beneficial effect of the Bath waters, they recover, their prospects are very little brightened: they feel no inclination, or perhaps ability, to engage in new pursuits; and if they are again employed in their old avocations, a return of the disease is sure to be the consequence, with the dreadful certainty, that the same remedies which relieved the first attack, will stand little chance of success on a recurrence of the disorder. Thus, in the manufactories of white lead, they will never engage a workman who has been once seized with the painter's colic, well knowing that irreparable loss of limbs must ensue. Indeed, so deleterious are the fumes of lead, that I am acquainted with a plumber's family, where the arms of the children were contracted almost from their birth.

Sir George Baker observes, "the best preservative of those poor people who are obliged to expose themselves to the action of this poison, is greasy, unctuous food. This is well known to those who work in lead mines; and it is a common practice of the most prudent among the painters to take some fat broth, butter, or oil, every morning before they begin their daily work." It is, probably, on this principle that castor oil is so much recommended as an aperient medicine for this malady.

The poison of lead may be taken into the system either by impregnation of the mineral with our food, or externally through the lungs or the absorbents, as is the case with those who sleep or remain in houses newly painted. A melancholy instance of this kind occurred a few years since to a very worthy tradesman of this city, who lost his life in consequence of sleeping and taking his meals in the house whilst it was painting. In this case, if I have been rightly informed, the meat was hung up in the pantry newly painted, and nothing imbibes the noxious quality of paint more rapidly than raw flesh.

Although the external application of lead in its metallic form, in a case quoted from Dr. Wall, produced palsy, yet I have never seen or heard of any injury being produced by the external use of the goulard lotion. It never has produced the slightest tendency to the complaint, even in those cases where it was applied on a most extended surface, and where there was every chance of absorption. A strong case in point I shall briefly mention. A few years ago, the man servant of Mr. Hopkins, in Marlborough-buildings in this city, whilst brewing, fancied he could be of more assistance by getting on the top of the boiler; whilst in this situation his feet slipped into the boiler. He was, of course, instantly taken out; but on cutting away his stockings, the whole skin peeled off from the knees to the toes. I immediately applied strong goulard water in the form of a bran poultice, constantly wetted, and though there were a few ulcerations rather tedious, yet, with this application solely, the man was able to walk about in three weeks. Had this application been likely to produce any deleterious effect, I think there could not have been a more favourable opportunity.

The mode in which the Bath waters are prescribed in this complaint is chiefly by bathing and pumping; the former three times in the week, according to the former directions; and the latter on the diseased limbs, and on the spine, to the amount of four or five hundred strokes every other day. Where there is considerable debility and want of tone in the stomach, the waters may be administered internally with the greatest advantage.

The Bath waters, though strongly recommended by physicians, both ancient and modern, in this species of paralysis, can only prove efficacious by a proper trial, the length of which must depend on the degree of improvement and the violence of the attack. On a reference to the cases admitted into the Hospital, it appears that some patients continued six months, others nine; and in more obstinate cases they will feel very little amendment in less than a year. But when the limbs begin to improve, then is the time to persevere, though many patients are eager to leave off the means, the moment the slightest advance is perceived.

The necessity of exertion, when once the slightest ability is felt, need not be enforced. All paralytics must second the use of the various remedies by every means in their power. Neglect of the bowels will often occasion a relapse of the complaint; and though the taking of medicine continually may be very unpleasant, yet it is much more unpleasant to be obliged to an assistant for every meal we wish to convey to our mouths.

The beneficial effects of the Bath waters cannot be more strongly pointed out, than by giving Dr. Charlton's account of these diseases admitted into the Bath Hospital during a period of thirteen years; which affords a more convincing proof, than all the idle theories can possibly subvert.

"Palsies from mineral effluvia, 40.—Cured and "benefited, 38; dead, and no better, 2.

"Palsies from cider and bilious colic, 237.—Cured "and benefited, 218; dead, and no better, 19."

From the able observations of Sir George Baker and Dr. Warren, also from the decided conviction of Dr. Andrew, of Exeter, from which county the greatest number of the cider and bilious cases were sent, it must be evident that all the above cases, though differently classed by Dr. Charlton, originated from the same cause; and it is but fair to take the aggregate of the whole, in estimating the superior virtues of the Bath waters. The above statement speaks volumes, and none but the wilfully blind will shut their senses against conviction.

These cases of paralysis are some of the most distressing, for which the virtues of the bathing and pumping are recommended; and the benefit derived is so strong and unequivocal, that no collusion or attempt to enhance their value can possibly be surmised. That they sometimes fail is most certain; but in general their failure arises either from the irregularity of the patient, or from the application of the bath having been deferred too long.

Dr. Warren relates the following anecdote of a whole family being seized with this disorder from the infamous practice of purifying white wine by means of lead; and there can be very little hesitation in believing the colic of Poitou, and many others, to originate from the same source.

In June, 1752, thirty-two persons in the Duke of Newcastle's family, then residing at Hanover, were seized with the *colica pictonum*, after having used as their common drink a small white wine, that had been adulterated with some of the calces of lead. As the complaint was not well understood when it first appeared, and the usual consequences of violent pains in the bowels with obstinate costiveness were apprehended, recourse was had to bleeding, clysters, and various kinds of purgatives, by which means every symptom was increased.

They were all attacked in the common way, excepting one, whose first seizure was an epileptic fit. As soon as the fit was over, he complained of pain in the bowels; and upon the ceasing of the pain in the bowels, his head was affected again; a disorder like St. Vitus's dance came on, and in less than a fortnight from the first attack he died epileptic.

Three were feverish from the beginning to the end of the disease. The rest were perfectly free from fever till the fourth or fifth day, at which time the pain began to abate, and their pulses became quicker than in health.

Some of them complained that their mouths and throats were made sore by the acrimony of the matter they vomited up. Four fell into salivations for several hours every day, and said that their pain was abated during the spitting. Many of them had profuse sweats just before the disorder terminated; and a few had an eruption of white and red pimples, which were very fiery, and itched exceedingly. One was delirious, and in that state was put into the warm bath, and recovered his senses while he was in the water, and at last got perfectly well.

All of them relapsed within four or five days after they seemed to have been cured. Many had the disorder thrice, and some few of them five times. It is very probable that the cause of the complaint was not discovered, nor a more wholesome drink provided, till some time after the disease appeared; but the relapses were supposed to have been caused by sudden exposition to wet and cold, or by intemperate eating.

The method of cure differed very little from that laid down above, except that a glyster of oil and brown sugar was injected every night, and a spoonful of oil of almonds, with two drachms of syrup of lemon juice, was directed to be taken every six hours. Their nourishment was barley broth, barley pudding, with currants and panada.

One of them had a severe return of the colic two years afterwards; he was cured by the method described above, and has remained well ever since. Another relapsed five years afterwards, has had nine returns of the colic since that time, and is now in the chronical state of the disease, with the fingers of both hands paralytic. It is remarkable that this person has never been free from costiveness since the attack in 1752, *except when under a course of Bath waters.*

One died of the colic, five have died since of other complaints, twenty-six are still alive, and only one of them has been rendered paralytic by the disorder.

Dr. Cooke relates the two following cases, one from lead and the other from arsenic, where the symptoms, he says, are nearly similar, but in the latter more violent.

A person a few years ago was admitted into St. Bartholomew's Hospital, under the care of Dr. Powell, who was affected with palsy from this cause in a very extraordinary degree. The patient, who was a painter, was totally regardless of cleanliness in his business, and was in the habit of wiping his brush on the sleeves of his coat, so that he was particularly exposed to the fumes of the paint which he used. In this case not only the hands of the patient were paralytic, but also the lower extremities, and the sphincter muscles of the bladder.

In the Medical and Physical Journal the case of a young man is related, who had been afflicted with paralysis of the upper and lower extremities, with violent pains in the muscles and bowels, produced by arsenic, which he had mixed with butter and wheat flour, and made into pills by rolling the composition in his hands. The disease, after some time, proved fatal. The symptoms resembled those produced by the poison of lead, but were more violent.

A few years since a Gentleman, about 60 years of age, holding a high situation in the War Office, came to Bath totally divested of the use of his hands and arms, and very much debilitated in his feet. This gentleman, from a sedentary life, had never enjoyed very good health; his digestive organs were bad, and biliary secretions uncertain. He never had any thing like paralysis of his limbs, until after his office was fresh painted. Not conceiving it could do him any injury, as soon as the paint was dry he repaired to his office as usual, and remained several hours every day. A few days after this circumstance he was seized with a violent attack in his bowels, and, from his own account, had a decided lead colic. On the relief of the bowels, he was seized with a paralysis of the upper extremities, and general debility of his whole frame. His legs, however, were not entirely useless, as he contrived to walk with them, but apparently with a great effort, as he threw his legs forward with a sudden jerk. As for his arms and wrists they were totally useless, and the hands with a disposition to turn inwards. He was subject to violent pains all over the body, and very disordered stomach, with confined bowels. The latter might partly be owing to a bad habit he had acquired of taking a large quantity of laudanum every night to relieve the pains. The first object was to diminish the laudanum, and induce the bowels to act. This with difficulty being accomplished, he began the Bath waters in all their forms, bathing, pumping, and drinking, and with some intermissions continued this course for nine months, when he went away so much better as to be able to write, and lift his hand to his mouth. After being absent from Bath some months, he returned and resumed the use of the waters with the greatest benefit. Nearly two years afterwards I saw this patient at his country house, perfectly recovered.

In the year 1811, the butler to a noble family came for the use of the waters in a case of dropped hands. It was not known how the disease originated; but he was seized with violent spasmodic twitchings and constipation of the bowels, which ultimately terminated in paralysis of the wrists. When he came to Bath, he had no particular disease, excepting the paralysis; his general health was good, but he suffered occasional pains in his arms and wrists, and great difficulty in keeping his bowels regular. The paralysis had continued five months without any amendment, notwithstanding various applications and medicines had been tried. As a last resource he came to Bath. He was put on a course of pumping and bathing, and after three months was so far relieved as to be able to open the door. His bowels were constantly acted upon by medicine, and he lived moderately. By degrees the wrists acquired strength, and the muscles their plumpness, and he left Bath very much benefited.

S. F. esq; a gentleman from Buckinghamshire, came to Bath in a very deplorable state in the month of July, 1819. He had entirely lost the use of his limbs, both hands and feet; was subject to violent spasms in his bowels, which the most powerful medicines would hardly relieve; likewise flying pains all over his limbs, and almost incessant vomiting. The muscles of the shoulder were very much diminished; and the state of exhaustion so great, that although he had a rapid quick pulse, he was obliged to be supported by brandy, laudanum, and æther.

This gentleman, about three months before his visit to Bath, had suffered severely in his health by exposure to cold, and checked perspiration; and in this weak state he unfortunately remained in his house in the country whilst it was painting. About ten days afterwards paralysis of the limbs came on gradually, attended with violent muscular pains and obstinate costiveness. The violent sufferings and the singularity of the attack induced this gentleman to remove to town for the benefit of further medical advice, where he was under the care of Sir Gilbert Blane; who tried a number of remedies, amongst the rest, mustard poultices to the wrists and feet. The Doctor likewise gave strong mercurial purgatives, which produced nothing but black fœtid motions. The patient daily getting worse, Sir Gilbert, in conjunction with Dr. Baillie, advised his coming to Bath; the former candidly acknowledging that he scarce expected he would reach it alive. Alive he did reach it; but a more deplorable case never was witnessed, and it was many weeks before his most sanguine friends had an idea that it was possible he could recover. It was, of course, some time before he could make trial of the waters: the first object was to preserve life by allaying spasm, quieting the vomiting, and acting on the bowels.

In this case the liver was very much deranged; and in the course of the cure, whenever the stomach was disordered, and the secretions not properly attended to, the progress of the limbs invariably retrograded. It was nearly six weeks before this gentleman could begin a very small glass of water, which he did with evident advantage; and he likewise used the bath, which was persevered in more regularly than the drinking, on account of the capricious state of the stomach and the torpor of the bowels. It would be endless to state the whole medical treatment in this case, which, of course, was obliged to be regulated by existing circumstances; but Dr. Robertson, who latterly attended this gentleman with myself, can bear testimony to the distressing symptoms and violence of the attack, and the little prospect there appeared of ultimate recovery. However, from a totally helpless state, and loss of motion in both extremities, by the constant use of the waters this gentleman left Bath in January, 1820, able to walk, and beginning to assist himself by the use of his hands.

This patient returned to Bath in January, 1821, and ever since that period to the present moment has occasionally used the waters; the consequence is, that he has the perfect use of hands and feet, although the muscles of the feet are a little contorted, and there is occasional debility of the wrists, whenever the bile is not properly secreted. As a strong argument in favour of bathing, it should be mentioned that this patient remains in the bath generally an hour, and sometimes an hour and a half, and always with advantage.

The most extraordinary part of this case deserves to be recorded—that none of the medical men at a distance suspected the disease to arise from the impregnation of lead; some attributing the loss of limbs to gout, others to bile; and one practitioner, supposing it to arise from the spine, blistered it from top to bottom. It would be very easy to prove, if our limits would allow, that twenty cases of paralysis would occur where one is now observable, if gout or bile could be deemed the cause.

The two following cases, extracted from Dr. Cooke's work on Palsy, are merely adduced to shew how powerfully the poison of lead acts on the human constitution; and to point out its deleterious effects from the slightest causes.

A Gentleman laboured under a paralytic affection of the whole of one side of his face, for which neither he nor any of his family could assign any probable cause. After numerous fruitless enquiries, I at last found, that for two or three nights he had slept in a room in which there was a closet, the door of which had been recently painted in what is called a dead white colour. His bed was placed close to this door; and as the weather was warm, he slept without curtains, that side of the face which afterwards became paralytic being turned towards the painted door. Under these circumstances, with the knowledge I had of the deleterious effects of lead in other cases, I had no hesitation in ascribing this partial palsy to the fumes arising from the paint.

Dr. Perceval in his Experiments and Observations mentions, from Dr. Wall, the case of a child, about two years of age, the son of a plumber, who had been always remarkably healthy, who was seized with violent pains in the bowels, attended with a fever and convulsive motions in the limbs. These complaints were attributed to worms; and several medicines had been unsuccessfully given. When Dr. Wall visited him first, he found him paralytic on one side, and delirious. "Upon enquiry "into the cause of his disorder, and particularly whe-"ther the child had been used to go into the room "where they melted the lead, he was informed that he "did frequently; and that it was a custom with his "maid to let him run barefooted along the sheets of "lead whilst they were warm, with which he appeared "to be much delighted." Dr. W. did not then hesitate to attribute the disorder to this cause.

We have quoted the two next cases from Dr. Pierce; they are decided cases of *colica pictonum*, and prove the particular benefit of the waters.

The Rev. Mr. P., aged 33, came hither for the use of the bath. He lived near the Fens; to which *uliginous* air was ascribed the beginning of his illness. After such a colic he was crippled and emaciated all over; his legs were in some measure recovered before he came hither, for he could walk, though but feebly, and had not much pain; but his arms and hands were wholly useless, and hung like flails; he could not lift either of them to his head, nor could he grasp any thing with his hands; the great muscles of the thumb (wherein chiefly consists the strength of the hand) were quite wasted. He could not feed himself, much less put off and on his own clothes. After preparatory purging, I put him upon drinking the waters to prevent the return of the colic, (for he had some threatenings of a recidivation,) and a chalybeate course, and bathing occasionally, as his weakness would bear it. The first proof of his being better, with much joy, to shew his improvement, coming to my house, he put off his hat to me; for though he was a Clergyman, his disease had made him so much a Quaker, that he could not perform that accustomed civility to any one, till after awhile bathing. Before he went hence he could write his name competently well, though he could not hold a pen for many months before. He staid six or seven weeks, and then went away greatly benefited. He returned the next year, and perfected what he had so well begun the year before.

The Right Hon. Nicholas Earl of T., aged between 50 and 60, came here very feeble in his limbs, but especially in his arms and hands; he had scarcely a muscle upon either left visible; and was not able to help himself in any respect. The ligaments at his shoulders were so relaxed, that his arms hung like flails, and he threw them forward and backward, rather than moved them; with this weakness of limbs, he had decay of appetite and digestion. He nauseated every thing, and was reduced even to a skeleton; and all this the effect of a bilious colic, which continued long upon him. After the translation of the matter to the nerves, he was, by fits, at ease in his bowels, but thus weakened in his limbs, for which he came to Bath. His Lordship drank the waters and bathed; took alteratives, aperients, and antiscorbutics; and by degrees got stomach, ease, and strength, but staid two or three months for it. His Lordship came several times after to confirm what he had at first attained.

The following cases we quote from Guidot; and though the origin of the complaints, and the cases altogether, are not very distinctly related, yet the characteristic marks are too decided to be mistaken.

Peter Bonamy, sub-dean of Guernsey, three years troubled with the colic, on a translation of the morbific matter to the limbs, became paralytic. There was also added a scorbutic taint, by which the mass of blood was defiled, and the animal spirits became languid and weak; the skin infested with spots and pustulous eruptions, the fingers contracted, feet staggering, and the internal muscular flesh of the right thumb very much sunk, with paleness of his countenance, and leanness over all the body. The first season of bathing in the temperate bath gave him considerable advantage in health in a month's time; the second season more; and after four years' absence, coming to Bath again the third time, he returned with an athletic habit of body, fleshy and brawny limbs, only the extremities of his hands and feet, especially the back of the foot, weak; otherwise sound; his bowels, as far as by touch and conjecture could appear, no way ill affected; and, the weakness before excepted, every where strong and sound. He used the King's and Queen's Bath chiefly, and sometimes the Cross Bath, and drank the water from the King's Bath dry-pump.

Mr. Moses Levermore, chirurgeon at Nevis, afflicted with the colic or belly-ache, which afterwards turned to the palsy; by the use of the King's and Cross Baths, but especially the Cross, received cure the 3d of September, 1686.

Elias Pomeroy, in the county of Devon, esq; having the same disease, and using the King's Bath little more than one month, found great benefit. He had also many times six hundred pumps from the dry pump on the weak hand. In both these persons the muscle at the root of the right thumb sunk very much, as observed in Peter Bonamy, sub-dean of Guernsey.

About the year 1640, a Welsh Gentleman, operator, concerned in the silver mines in Wales, was stricken with a poisonous steam, to the loss of use of all his limbs, in the place where they wrought; and presently coming in a coach to Bath, was advised by Dr. Bave, an old eminent physician, then practising at that place, to the use of the King's Bath; where, by the help of bathing, and the scum of the bath applied to the parts affected, in the nature of a poultice, in a month's time he could stand and walk a little, and in three months' time was so well recovered, that he could go without the help of a staff, and ride a mettled horse home well. He was cured in one season of bathing.

A Youth, about 19 years of age, who two years ago was seized with a West-India colic, after a voyage to those parts, was admitted a patient here in September last, and was the most miserable object ever beheld. His arms hung entirely useless by his sides, the hands dropped quite inwards, greatly emaciated, and the fingers so strongly contracted, that it was not in the power of force to move them; the legs were so wasted as to appear only covered with skin, and contracted up to his buttocks, so that he always stood on his knees. This lad, by the use of bathing, soon began to recover, and has been for some time able to walk without crutches; he has now the free use of his hands, the legs and arms are become plump, and the flexor muscles of the thumbs have nearly regained their size, though they were more wasted than I ever saw.*

The following seven interesting cases and remarks I have extracted from Dr. Charlton's tracts.

* Summers on Paralysis, page 28.

They are part of the evidence of the hospital practice in proving the efficacy of the Bath waters in this most distressing complaint. That they all had their origin from the impregnation of *lead* there can be little doubt, and some of the cases are most interesting, as pointing out how slight an exposure to this deleterious poison is capable of affecting the constitution. In many cases which I have seen, and in similar ones related both by Drs. Guidot and Pierce, it is very evident, that a repetition of these attacks is seldom benefited in the same degree (if at all) by the use of the waters.

William Bishop, of Dunster, in Somersetshire, of a spare habit of body, was affected with an excruciating pain in his stomach, which, soon extending to the bowels, brought on a total obstruction, that continued for ten days. These complaints were occasioned by his having drank freely of cider. A passage being at length procured, the pains in his stomach and bowels in some degree abated; whereupon a weakness seized his wrists, and gradually deprived him of the use of both hands, the backs of which were covered with large hard tumours, that for a time were extremely painful. It was a year and nine months from the time this person first lost the use of his hands, before he was sent to Bath. The hands fell pendulous from the wrists, the power of raising them being gone. The fingers were contracted into the palms of the hands, and could not be extended. Except the affection of these parts, he was in other respects well, his bowels having long been free from obstruction. After a few doses of physic, he drank the waters, and went into the bath. When he had bathed about a fortnight, he was ordered to have his hands pumped every day, and by these means he in a very few weeks was entirely cured.

It is to be observed that five or six other persons belonging to the same place were affected about the same time, and from the like cause, in their stomach and bowels, which terminated in a palsy of their limbs; and that they were all, together with this patient, discharged from the Bristol Infirmary without having received any benefit, but were afterwards perfectly recovered by the Bath waters.

John Holman, by drinking too freely of cider, when heated with labour, was attacked with a colic, which lasted five weeks, and was accompanied with a constipation of the bowels, fever, and delirium. As soon as his costiveness was removed, the fever and delirium left him, and the pains in his bowels were much abated. On the remission of these pains his knees began to swell; but these swellings soon subsiding, his hands became paralytic, and then his bowels grew perfectly easy. This palsy of the hands did not continue above a month; the disease gradually abated of itself, till it entirely left him. The next year, from the like indiscretion, his disorder returned, and was attended with the same symptoms; which having lasted longer than on the first attack, in the end totally destroyed the action of his arms and hands. In this condition, near seven months after his relapse, he came to the Hospital. He drank the waters, bathed, and was pumped, and in a couple of months regained the perfect action and strength of his arm; but the muscles of the fingers not advancing equally in their recovery with those of the arms, blisters were applied to the wrists, by which these parts were also restored to their natural powers. He was admitted a patient the 9th February, 1760, and was discharged the 28th of May.

Nicholas Neale was taken with a colic, attended with a diarrhœa, upon drinking some new cider; which complaints continued for fourteen weeks. He then found his voice begin to faulter, and for some days could not speak to be understood. After this, his speech returned; and then his arms and hands became paralytic. These limbs hung loose and helpless from the trunk of the body, and were affected with severe pains continually running from the ends of his fingers to the points of his shoulders. In this state he was received into the Hospital the 1st of April, 1759; and by the customary methods was perfectly cured by the 18th July. I have been induced to mention this case from a circumstance attending it, which is contrary to the usual progress of the disease. For though a purging came on at the beginning of the seizure, and continued till the colic ceased, yet a palsy first seized the organs of voice, and then shifting to the arms and hands entirely took away their use.

Lead, we know, is remarkably productive of this complaint. The *sugar of lead* has been recommended in some cases as medicinal, and, perhaps, when judiciously used, may have proved so; but when given internally, or applied externally, without proper caution, it is found to bring on the disease. The same effect is produced by correcting acid wines with *sugar of lead;* and a similar instance, not long since, fell under my own knowledge, of six persons who became at the same time paralytic by drinking cider brought to them while at harvest work in a new earthen pitcher, whose inside was glazed; which glazing is made chiefly of *lead*, and was undoubtedly dissolved by the cider, as appeared not only from the unhappy effects which drinking it produced, but also from its having given (as these persons informed me) that astringent sweetish taste to the liquor, by which solutions of this mineral are peculiarly distinguished.

Allen Lane, of Portbury, in Somersetshire, mariner, aged 19, was in the year 1749, attacked in the West-Indies with the dry belly-ache, which brought on a fever, convulsions, and loss of senses. These complaints continued for some time; and upon their quitting him, he was entirely deprived of the use of all his limbs. It was near a twelvemonth after this paralytic seizure before he came to England, and was, at my recommendation, admitted into the hospital, under the care of the late Dr. Sommers. His arms hung useless, like flails, from his body; his fingers were drawn into the palms of his hands, the backs of which were covered with large hard swellings. His legs were contracted close to his buttocks, and so fixed there, that no external force could displace them. In consequence of this contraction, which made it impossible for him to put his feet to the ground, he rested on his knees; and when he was to remove from one place to another, it was done by crawling on them and his elbows. The muscles of the whole body were greatly emaciated, particularly those of the arms and legs. His bowels were excessively costive, and frequently tormented with pains; he was often sick at his stomach, and had little or no appetite. The first intention in this case was to get the stomach and bowels into a natural state by improving the appetite and digestion, and procuring a free passage for the excrements. These points were at length effected by a proper regimen of diet, the occasional use of mild aperient medicines, and the waters drank in small quantities. He now became able to venture on bathing, and to make use of the pump; which measures he continued till his stay in the hospital was no longer necessary.

It may easily be imagined that it required a long use of these waters, before a disease of such inveteracy could be expected to give way to them; but it at last yielded, in a great measure, to their powers, though not till he had resided here 622 days.

He was discharged the 20th of May, 1752, minuted in our register, *Much better*. For his general health was in all respects restored; the contraction of his legs was entirely removed; their muscles were grown fleshy and full; and the complete action of the lower limbs was regained. He had also the use of his arms and hands; but the muscles of these parts, particularly of the latter, were still weak and emaciated; and it is most probable they never recovered their natural strength and size, as I do not remember more than one or two instances where a complete atrophy had once possessed the muscles of the hands, especially those which form the ball of the thumb, that the parts ever recovered their natural fulness and strength.

It seems extremely probable that this attack must have arisen from some mineral impregnation.

Thomas Woodden, painter of earthen ware, was twice admitted into *St. Thomas's Hospital* for a colic and palsy, which were the effects of his occupation, and was both times much relieved; but still so great a weakness remained in his wrists, as to render him incapable of using his hands; on which account he was sent to our Hospital, where he was perfectly recovered in one hundred and forty days. We have a great number of instances of this kind on our books, but this case I have particularly selected, as it shews that a very small quantity of that noxious mineral, *lead,* (for very little, I am informed, is used in the business which this man followed,) is capable of producing the most pernicious effects. Happy would it be if some other pigment could be discovered, which might supply its place; for even the very effluvia which arises from newly painted houses has sometimes proved as hurtful to the inhabitants, as mixing the colours and laying them on too commonly prove to the painters themselves.

Samuel Butts, aged 41, of St. George's, Hanover-square, of a thin habit of body, and pale complexion, was seized with colic pains in his bowels, attended with a little quickness of pulse and costiveness, about the 20th of August, 1753. Proper means were used to relieve him, by the advioe of a very experienced physician. Notwithstanding all the assistance that could be given him, his pains continued about three weeks, sometimes very violent, at others more gentle; but he was never during that period free from them. As they began to abate, he gradually had a weakness of his legs and arms come on, which has increased so much in his arms and wrists as to disable him from feeding or dressing himself, and has reduced him to a very helpless condition. During the whole time of the complaint, stools have been with great difficulty procured. He lived in a house while it was new painted, when taken ill.

This patient, whose complaints were exactly similar to those which painters themselves so often suffer, came into our hospital October 15th, 1753, and was discharged cured the May following.

Edward Erridge, of Willington, in Sussex, aged 29, by trade an optic-glass maker, which business he had followed for near twenty years without any inconvenience, was one day very suddenly taken, as he was grinding glass, with a most violent spasmodic pain in his stomach, and continual vomiting; to which ensued so costive a state of body, that he was frequently for a fortnight together without any evacuation, during which time the pains he felt in his belly were intolerable. For these complaints, together with wandering pains that more particularly affected his arms, he was admitted into *Guy's Hospital*; where he found, with respect to the disorder in his bowels, a good deal of benefit, and was advised by his physician to repair to Bath for the completion of his cure. But not following this advice, he continued for some months in a miserable condition, from the pains which had now fixed together in his arms, but which at length gradually wore away, and were succeeded by a paralytic shaking of these limbs. In this state he continued for five months; when the tremblings ceased, and he lost the use of both his hands. He came to our Hospital March 14th, 1752; and was discharged in the August following, much better. He returned to us again in December, pursued the same course of bathing and pumping till the 5th of April, when he obtained a perfect cure.

I find by Dr. Oliver's papers, he was informed by a patient, who was paralytic in his arm from the same cause as the person whose history is above related, that from the wheel used in grinding glass, which is turned by a rapid water course, there is frequently emitted a blue flame, which smells very sulphureous, and is so excessively poisonous, that many who follow this business grow consumptive, some lose their senses, but the generality are subject to colics, which usually terminate in palsies of the hands. The person who gave the Doctor this information laboured under the latter complaint; of which he was cured by the Bath waters in two hundred and fifty-one days, but relapsed by returning to his business, and upon a re-admission into the Hospital received no benefit.

Painters, refiners, gilders, and all who are employed in digging ore, or in the separation of the metals from it, are liable to colics, which end in palsies. The symptoms are much the same with those which proceed from cider, and the Bath waters are equally a remedy, by which ever of these causes the disease is produced ; with this difference, however, that palsies from mineral effluvia require the longest use of the waters to effect their cure.

It is apparent from these cases, that the patients usually recommended to our Hospital labour under palsies which have resisted the powers of medicine, and whose original obstinacy has, of course, been augmented by time ; yet the table informs us, that out of nine hundred and sixty-nine paralytics, in situations so unpromising, eight hundred and thirteen were benefited.

It cannot have escaped the reader's notice, that *bathing* in these waters makes an essential part in the hospital practice.

We bathe all our paralytics, where no particular circumstances forbid. When a patient is sent hither, whose limbs, from a long continuance of the disease are totally relaxed, warm immersion in such a state would be manifestly improper ; and he is, there, obliged to refrain, till by drinking the waters, or, if necessary, by the aid of medicine, he requires a sufficient degree of strength to venture on its use. Where no such objections occur, he enters on this course after a short preparation. If the bath weaken, as it sometimes does, he intermits it; and in the mean time has his limbs pumped. Some are able both to bathe and pump at the same time, or else to use each alternately; while others stand in need of pumping alone; and thus the external application of the waters is prevalent in all such complaints, though varied according to the particular nature of the case, and the constitution of the patient.

Should the curious reader now want to know after what manner the Bath waters act in the cure of paralytic diseases, his first solicitude should be employed in seeking how animal motion and sensation arise from the brain and nerves. That these organs are necessary to the performance of the animal functions is well known; but how they perform them remains yet, and is likely to remain, an inexplicable secret. While nature, therefore, so industriously conceals from us the *manner* of her operations, it should teach us to confine our studies to the acquirement of that useful knowledge, which is the fruit of patient attention to their *consequences* and *effects,* instead of pursuing speculations, and forming systems, which, when well founded, have proved of little use in the art of healing; and when ill founded, a positive hindrance to our progress in it.

INDIGESTION, OR DYSPEPSIA.

In our observations on gout, rheumatism, and palsy, we have plainly evidenced, as far as proof can go, the superior benefit derived in these disorders from the *external* application of the Bath waters; and now we proceed to demonstrate, that in no class of disease is their *internal* exhibition more decisively advantageous, and as such more generally acknowledged, than in cases of indigestion, or affections of the stomach.

Indigestion can seldom be considered an idiopathic disease, but is generally symptomatic of some derangement of the system.

It is a complaint very difficult to be clearly defined; it may, however, be distinguished by nausea, loss of appetite, eructations of various kinds, distension of the stomach and bowels, heart-burn, gnawing pain in the region of the stomach, food frequently thrown up many hours after taken in an undigested state, inconstant state of the bowels, general debility, &c.; and these symptoms frequently accompanied by great depression and lowness of spirits. The head often suffers from sympathy, and the eyes are affected with dimness, and spots appearing between the sight and the object; the latter is also a common incident in bilious affections. These symptoms, however, do not always occur in the same patient, but vary according to the exciting cause.

Its causes are various. It may proceed from organic disease, such as tumours, ulcers, or schirrosity of the stomach; but it more generally arises from excesses in living, long fasting, sedentary occupations, too close application to study, &c. As for tea or coffee producing this disease, I do not believe it to be the case; were we to dilute more, indigestion would be less frequent. It may also be symptomatic of gout, pregnancy, worms, or, indeed, any general derangement of the system.

Dr. Wilson Philip arranges the symptoms of indigestion under three stages. The first stage, such symptoms as arise from undigested food, or an overloaded stomach, such as flatulence, distention, and eructations, &c.; from a recurrence of which symptoms the viscera become changed, and the secretions disordered, producing feverish thirst, impaired appetite, bilious fæces, general debility, and irregular circulation.

The second stage is marked by great tenderness, on pressure of the right side, between the pit of the stomach and bend of the ribs, with considerable increase of fever. This tenderness Dr. Philip ascribes to an inflammatory state of the pylorus, and of the thin edge of the liver that lies over it, and is in contact with it.

The third is that stage of indigestion, which, from long continuance and aggravated returns, is eventually productive of organic disease.

Indigestion, or an improper assimilation of the food, either from its quantity or quality, may exist for a considerable time without materially disordering the system; but a continual recurrence of these slight attacks of flatulence and acid eructations will at length produce an alteration in the secretions, and a long train of those distressing symptoms which are their natural consequence.

The first attacks are generally removed without much trouble, (nature principally performing the office of physician;) but, like the gout and many other diseases, the oftener it recurs, the more difficult it becomes to relieve the distressing debility and the relaxed state of the stomach.

Where this disease arises from any organic affection, our means are very confined, the symptoms cannot be removed without a removal of the cause, which is generally beyond the reach of art. Where, however, it arises, as is most commonly the case, from our own imprudence, from the stimulus of high exciting food, which forces the energies of the stomach beyond its tone, in such case our first object should be to correct the irregularities of diet, and endeavour to restore the weakened action of the stomach by proper remedies.

The medicines usually recommended in this complaint are those which have a tendency to strengthen the stomach, such as bitters and chalybeate waters, correcting the acidity by magnesia and alkalis, taking moderate exercise, attention to the bowels, and avoiding high-seasoned food or strong drinks.

There must, however, be great discrimination with regard to diet in the treatment of patients labouring under stomach complaints. A difference must, of course, be observed between those cases arising from constitutional debility and others the consequence of high excitement. Solid food of the plainest kind may be observed as a general direction, and a little brandy and water may in some cases be allowed with advantage; but wine, beer, and all fermenting liquors should be voided.

The use of the Bath water is, however, most beneficial, when bitters, food, and every thing else taken into the stomach have been rejected. It warms and comforts the stomach, acts as a gentle stimulant and bracer to the relaxed fibres, and promotes that natural appetite, which has been so long a stranger to the dyspeptic patient.

The bathing, likewise, at the temperature of from 94° to 96°, soothes the nervous irritability which usually accompanies this class of patients. Besides these remedies, if strict attention be paid to the diet, with gentle evacuant medicines, and horse exercise, if the patient can bear it, he will soon feel the benefit of his perseverance.

Sir George Gibbes bears ample testimony to the benefit dyspeptic patients derive from both the internal and external use of the Bath waters; and Dr. Falconer observes, that "every medical practitioner at this place has seen instances of people "labouring under want of appetite, pain, and "spasm of the stomach and bowels, together with "all the other symptoms of depraved digestion, "and want of power in the proper organs to perform their functions, joined to a very great degree "of weakness, both of the body and of the spirits, "relieved by the use of the Bath waters. The "recovery in such cases is particularly remarkable "for its taking place so quickly after the commencement of the trial of the remedy. A few "days will frequently work such a change in the "situation of the patient as would be scarcely credible, were it of less common occurrence. The "appetite is often restored altogether, the wandering spasms and pain cease, the natural rest

" returns, and the spirits are raised to their proper " pitch. The strength likewise improves daily, " and the natural secretions and regularity of the " body in point of evacuations are restored."

In all weakness of the organs of digestion, or want of tone in the muscular fibres of the stomach, whether arising from the too frequent use of strong liquors, or general indulgence in the luxuries of the table, the Bath waters have, no doubt, the most beneficial effect. But it is only by a determination to abstain from these irregular habits and powerful exciting causes of dyspepsia, that any permanent benefit can be expected. A return to Bath wine instead of Bath water will most certainly, sooner or later, bring on organic disease either of the stomach or the liver, or else occasion a tendency to plethora, which will be equally decisive as to its result.

We should likewise consider how many other diseases are brought on by intemperance in eating and drinking, and want of exercise. The sufferings of dyspeptic patients in aggravated cases are tolerably severe ; but what are they, compared to the gout, stone, scurvy, apoplexy, cancers, dropsies, &c.? some one of these being the invariable termination of long continued debility of the digestive organs. Were it possible for young men, whilst plunging into every scene of vice and dissipation, to be in possession of the glass of

Lao,* and take a perspective view of all these diseases, whilst drinking "another and another "glass," they would be very apt to stop short in their career, and not barter an age of suffering for a few hours of apparent (not real) gratification.

Dr. Baynard, in alluding to the neglect with which young men treat a good constitution, and run into every excess of living, to the ruin of their health, has used some very forcible, though not very elegant, language on the occasion. He observes, "this supine and stupid neglect arises "from our too much trust in a good constitution; "when, alas, they think not that the least de-"bauch (though it does not blow up yet) like an "earthquake shakes the very foundation of the "human fabric, and repeated acts soon ruin the "superstructure. And because they see some few "old drunkards of fourscore safe waded through "an *aceldama* of their neighbours' skulls, that has "fallen in the battle, young men presently take "*non causa pro causa*, and imitate them in "drinking; not considering that this their prece-"dent, had he trimmed his lamp, and wisely "managed the flame, he might have lived to have "been an *Old Parr* or a *Jenkins*, &c. But, alas, "where one claret professor lives to eighty, ten "thousand of their tyros sink under it. I must "confess that company is very pleasant and charm-

* Goldsmith.

"ing, especially if it be all of a piece, witty and "ingenious; but we should consider how dearly "we purchase a little frothy and fleeting dis- "course," &c.

If, however, there are great numbers who bring this disorder on themselves by self-gratifications, there are likewise many, who, confined by business, or from hereditary disposition or constitutional debility, are, from their sufferings, very much to be pitied. To such, we are convinced, the Bath waters, under proper management, will afford the greatest relief; and if the disease has arisen from sedentary occupations, moderate and regular exercise should be observed, particularly horse exercise.

The stomach, likewise, should not be too long empty; a little food and often will benefit a weak stomach much more than long abstinence and a full meal; indeed, one cause of this complaint with many patients is long fasting, particularly with those engaged in business. Whatever, therefore, may be discovered to be the cause of dyspepsia, whether from full living, want of exercise, &c. it must be counteracted by a diametrically opposite system.

The food recommended as the easiest of digestion for weak stomachs is principally fresh beef and mutton, in preference to veal or lamb; poultry, game, and fish, may also be taken, as affording less nutriment; but hard salted meats should be avoided. Mealy potatoes are the best vegetable; greens of all kinds being acescent and flatulent. As every remedy has its day, so it is as liable to undergo a change in public opinion as the change of the fashions; thus with many of our brethren it is the fashion to advise no fluid to be drunk during meals, for fear of its diluting the gastric juice, and arresting the progress of nature in the digestive process. It is only astonishing how the machine works at all, when the wheels from such slight causes are so apt to be deranged, and when in addition to these dangers are considered those arising from the want of chemical affinity, it is more than wonderful we ever reach the grand climacteric!!

To be serious, we should advise patients labouring under difficulty of digestion *to avoid every kind of food which from experience disagrees;* and as every one is allowed to be a fool or a physician at forty, on this occasion we will allow them to be their own physician.

It is only in the chronic stage of this disease that the waters can be at all advised; when accompanied with inflammatory symptoms, they are prejudicial. When the bowels are well relieved, and the pulse is not quick, although the tongue may be white, it is no objection to the trial of the waters; for a white tongue is often symptomatic only of deranged digestion, and as the tone of the stomach is restored, the tongue acquires its natural appearance.

As the biliary secretions and other viscera are apt to be disordered in cases of indigestion, it is highly necessary that the state of the excretions should be particularly attended to; for the waters will require the occasional assistance of those medicines which are principally adapted for the removal of such obstructions.

It is inattention to the above circumstances in the early stages of indigestion which imperceptibly leads on to what Dr. Philip calls the third stage, or actual disease or schirrus of the liver, which usually terminates in dropsical affusion. Thus a disorder, which, in its first approaches, has nothing fatal or even very terrific in its appearance, and which by timely caution would soon be relieved, is gradually hurried on to a most formidable and incurable malady by imprudent excesses, and neglect of medical advice.

The mind should, likewise, be kept cheerful and amused, as depression of spirits generally accompanies dyspeptic patients. Thus, after a course of the Bath waters, which generally relieves the immediate symptoms, a change of scene presenting new objects will restore the mental energy, and gradually produce that concord between the stomach and the brain, which is so decidedly marked, that when the one organ becomes disordered, a sympathy of the other invariably takes place.

There are some other affections closely connected with indigestion, to which we shall briefly allude, particularly *hypochondriasis*, or low spirits, and *pyrosis*, or water brash. We shall, however, first give a few cases to shew the superior benefit of the Bath waters in all derangements of the organs of digestion.

The following six cases are extracted from Dr. Charlton and Dr. Oliver's memoranda: the five first are hospital cases, and speak decidedly in favour of the waters. Stomach complaints are not so frequent amongst the lower classes of the community; and when they do occur, they are not attended with the distressing dejection of spirits which afflicts the higher orders of society.

Ann Ashworth, of the parish of St. Bride's, London, is about 25 years of age; is a maid servant at present, but from her illness is incapable of doing her business. Her disorder is a violent pain at her stomach, with which she has been afflicted for the best part of five years, being seldom free from it above three or four weeks together; she has taken almost all kind of medicines usually administered in such cases, but has found only a temporary relief from them. We hope the Bath waters will be of service to her, and esteeming her a proper object of charity, recommend her to your Hospital. D. C. M. D.

Discharged cured, having been a patient 98 days.

Jane Walker, spinster, about 28 years of age, of a thin cold habit, has been for a long time subject to a violent pain in her stomach, attended with frequent irritations to vomit, so as not to keep any thing in her stomach; sometimes free of that complaint, but then violent gripings in her bowels without costiveness; the cause I presume to proceed from a weakness of the digestive faculty. All the means that have been used for her recovery have proved unsuccessful; and I humbly conceive that the waters would be of service to her.

J. Y.

Discharged cured, having been a patient 149 days.

William Collins, of Butleigh, has for some time laboured under a dangerous disorder, which Bath waters seem to me likely to remove. I apprehend there is some obstruction in the passage from the stomach to the duodenum. What suggests this conjecture is, that as soon as he has taken the smallest quantity of any solid food it gives him the most excruciating pains in his stomach, till it comes up again. And lately, if he eats any thing more substantial than broth, his stomach immediately swells like a blown bladder, and his breath is almost gone. S. H.

He was discharged cured, having been a patient 72 days.

This patient was 30 years of age. About three years before he came to Bath he caught a severe cold, and from that time was more or less troubled with indigestion, flatulency, and pain in the stomach. By degrees the pain of his stomach became more constant and more violent; to this was added an excessive degree of costiveness. No solid food staid in his stomach; he kept down broth better than any other nourishment, but even that he frequently flung up. About a quarter of a year before his admittance into our Hospital he began to discharge a clear insipid rheum from his mouth, which ran off to the quantity of four or five pints every twenty-four hours. He was much weakened and emaciated, and seemed falling into a hectic. He was prepared for the waters by a strong warm stomach purge He began to drink them in small quantities: they sat easy on his stomach, and in three days his vomiting was removed. The quantity of the waters was gradually increased, till he drank three half-pints of them in the day. He grew regular as to stools, and the discharge of the rheum from his mouth gradually decreased. He left the hospital perfectly free from all his complaints.

Solomon de Mattos, aged 54, was recommended to Bath for a stomach complaint. His case was similar to the preceding one, and was of near three years standing. His digestion was greatly impaired. He had continual retchings, in which he frequently discharged large quantities of a thin transparent humour. At times he had accessions of a hectic fever. This latter symptom made it dubious whether he should be allowed to drink the waters. But on the supposition that his fever might originate from inanition, he was allowed to try them, and in seventy days they completed his cure. Bath waters are usually forbid when feverish symptoms appear; but there can be no general rules without their exceptions. If the feverish symptoms are owing to an inflammatory state of the fluids, or from matter, drinking these waters would certainly destroy the patient; but when nervous debility occasions fever, they may, if taken with due caution, produce very happy effects, of which these two cases are sufficient proofs.

Elizabeth Vickers, about 46 years of age, has for several months complained of great pain in and about the stomach, which pains were often accompanied with eructations and vomitings.

It seems, that prior to these complaints she was subject to recurrent pains in her feet, which occasioned a suspicion that the symptoms above mentioned were of a gouty kind. Agreeably to this hypothesis the case was treated with warm purges, cardiacs, and stomachic medicines; but after a long pursuit of this method, no gouty paroxysm appearing, and, indeed, little or no benefit arising to the patient, excepting those short temporary reliefs which all warm spirituous compositions occasion in common, it was judged proper to direct saponaceous and aloetic medicines, which were afterwards followed by a course of aromatic bitters and chalybeats. This latter pursuit seemed to avail the patient considerably, but nevertheless was far from effecting a cure; for the pain, sickness, &c. every now and then returned, although not so severe as formerly, either as to degree or duration.

She was discharged cured, having been a patient 95 days.

After a proper preparation this woman was put upon a course of the waters; she continued drinking them for near a month without their producing any sensible alteration in her complaints. About this time she complained of great sickness, attended with a sensation of weight and load at her stomach; an emetic was given her, and she brought up more than a pint of thick black bile. After this discharge she sensibly found the waters do her good; her appetite mended, her digestion became perfect, and her evacuations regular. She was discharged relieved of all her complaints, without having had any gouty paroxysm to assist in their removal.

Mrs. Griffith was a lady well known, and by her great good-nature, and continual flow of cheerful spirits, much beloved and caressed by all who knew her. About 35 years since, great anxiety of mind threw her into a diarrhœa, followed by an entire loss of appetite, perpetual nausea, and vomitings up of every thing she attempted to get into her stomach. The great Dr. Friend was her physician; but the disease was too obstinate even for his skill to conquer. Tired with taking medicines, and finding herself grow worse, she, by the advice of some friends, asked the Doctor whether the Bath waters might not be serviceable in her case. The Doctor, tired as much as his patient by so long and fruitless an attendance, readily acquiesced in her making the trial, but without any very favourable prognostic of the success. She no sooner began to drink the waters than she felt her stomach and bowels mended by them; her symptoms were all relieved; the looseness grew very moderate; she took down food and digested it; and after drinking the waters about five or six weeks, she returned to London in such health, strength, and spirits, that her friends received her with joy and surprise. The benefit she found from this first Bath journey lasted a year and a half; when, from what cause I do not recollect, her bowels began to be out of order, and all her former complaints returned. Whither should she fly, but to the waters which had done her so much good when in the same circumstances? I was then in London, and came down with her in her own coach to Bath. I was then an eye witness of her miserable circumstances; the diarrhœa was violent; the vomiting as constant as ever she attempted to swallow any thing, either food or physic, except a spoonful now and then of brandy burnt on a lump of sugar, which staid in her stomach, and was almost her only support. As soon as we reached Bath she made all possible haste to the pump, and I saw her drink off a middling glass of the water with an eagerness and joy which we may form the justest idea of from the figures in Poussin's charming picture of Moses striking the Rock. The miracle was almost as great. She drank another glass, and declared that she felt herself quite well. From that hour she took down food, retained, and digested it; the looseness became moderate, and her spirits rose a degree or two above temperate. Having drunk the waters the usual time, she returned to London in good health, and remained so for many months; but by the next year she felt some admonitions from her stomach and bowels, to put her in mind that she ought to have recourse to her great remedy before she was driven to it by a total return of her complaints. She did so, and with the same success. But her constitution was too delicate, and her frame too much shattered by illness, to, be capable of being restored to strong or lasting health; yet by the help of Bath waters she lived a most comfortable, sprightly valetudinarian all the rest of her days. Many years she divided between this place and London, when she often enjoyed pretty long intervals of ease; but as soon as her stomach or bowels put her in mind of her former sufferings, she flew to the Bath waters, which never failed immediately to charm away her disorders. As she grew older and more infirm, she found herself become less and less capable of bearing any long absence from her great restorative, and that her London journeys were more and more fatiguing, as she was less able to bear their inconveniences. She therefore made this place her fixed habitation for the future. Here she spent her days in social pleasures, among her numerous friends, never omitting her visits to the pump, from which she received her daily support, and nobody was ever more sensible of, or more thankful for, the inestimable blessing. During some years before her death she took very little food; and if she did not keep her stomach alive by the waters, she could take none at all, but began to nauseate the sight and smell of victuals, till she could get a glass of the water as hot as possible, which alone could enable her to eat a mouthful. Thus by continually pouring a little oil into the lamp of life, though it burnt dimly, it did not quite go out until the seventy-sixth year of her age.

Mrs. B.'s case was so deplorable, through a weak and decayed stomach, of long standing, that she loathed every thing she either smelt or saw; and so weak and feeble she could scarcely stand. She vomited up every thing she took, whether liquids or solids, and melancholy to a strange degree, and emaciated to skin and bone. She took little or no rest, her pulse hardly perceptible, her eyes sunk; often eructations, and sometimes colic pains, accompanied with hysteric and splenetic fits, and generally clammy cold sweats on her head, face, arms, and hands; insomuch that she and all her servants thought she could not live a week. Being sent for to her, and finding her so extremely weak, and under such a general disorder of the whole frame, I considered that this was my Lady L.'s case exactly; who, when the vital flame was even blinking in the socket, and the soul (one foot over the threshold) turning out of its tattered and decayed tenement, by the cautious use of the Bath waters and bitters had a new life put to lease, and to this day enjoys an uninterrupted state of health. This lady was so very weak, that at first we gave her but two or three spoonfuls of the Bath water, and about half an hour after one spoonful of a bitter infusion; an hour after that a little more Bath waters, then bitters again; and so by degrees from less to more, I brought her to bear half a pint of the water hot from the pump, which staid without loathing or vomiting. Then she began to be reconciled to the sight and smell of meats, and to take a little chicken broth, &c.; and in a day or two more she could bear a pint taken at two or three draughts, and then began to eat solid meats, and in the space of nine or ten weeks recovered her health to admiration; insomuch, that when she went to church, or to walk in the Grove, when she came out of her chair she was pointed at, saying, There she is! that's she! that's the lady that was so weak! *Digito monstrare et dicier hæc est.*

Hypochondriasis,

Usually called Vapours or Low Spirits.

This is a disease more commonly affecting elderly than young people; and from many of its symptoms, and the deranged state of the viscera, may be considered a species of dyspepsia.

In addition, however, to the general symptoms of dyspepsia, this disease is distinguished by great languor, and want of resolution and activity; a disposition to seriousness, gloom, and timidity; and a great apprehension of the worst as to all future events. Such patients are particularly attentive to the state of their own health, and from the slightest morbid feelings apprehend the greatest danger. This despondency is often accompanied by pains about the left hypochondrium, with palpitation of the heart, general inquietude, and restless nights.

Its causes are similar to those producing dyspepsia, such as excesses in living, &c. but more particularly from anxiety of mind, or intemperance in study, which by degrees disorder the stomach, vitiate the secretions, weaken the energies of the brain, and gradually overturn the strongest intellectual fabric.

The only apprehension in this complaint is that from long continuance or a perseverance in the exciting cause, it may terminate in organic disease. If prudently managed, our prognosis is generally favourable.

The remedies advised in cases of indigestion are equally applicable in this complaint for the relief of the occasional symptoms; and when the patient is free from plethora, or fever, the use of the Bath waters, both external and internal, as recommended in dyspepsia, will be resorted to with the greatest benefit.

As, however, there is always great visceral derangement, emetics should be directed to clear the stomach, and mercurial medicines given to promote a proper secretion of the bile, and regularly persevered in until the appearances are perfectly natural, the liver being invariably more or less disordered in all cases of hypochondriasis. These precautions should be used previous to a trial of the waters; and even during their course the same means must be pursued to prevent bilious accumulations, to which there is always a tendency, and without the removal of which the waters would certainly do injury.

This is a disease which fortunately seldom affects the lower classes of society; yet it is melancholy to reflect, that some of the greatest characters the world has produced, have been the victims of its attacks. It undoubtedly arises, however, more frequently from mental than from sensual irregularity.

We do not consider hypochondriasis to be a disease of the mind, independent of bodily ailment; and indeed there are few cases of mental derangement which are not attributable to deranged functions of the stomach or the liver, and which may not be ultimately cured by a steady and persevering attention to those points. At the same time, however, that medicinal means are used for the removal of this species of despondency, moral treatment may be necessary, and a soothing, kind manner will gain the confidence of the patient, and materially assist the endeavours of the medical attendant.

Change of air and scene have been much recommended in this disorder; but it is not merely change of place which can cure the hypochondriac patient, if the mind be not roused at the same time—some *hobby* to be indulged in, some pursuit to be relished, will alone relieve the depression of spirits, which, without some resource, will accompany the wanderer "from Indus to the Pole."

From the above observations it is but candid to acknowledge, that neither Bath waters, nor any other remedy, can be of much service without calling to our aid employment and amusement for the mind. Not that employment which brings a host of cares with it, and which probably has proved the cause of the malady, but rational amusement, varied with judgement, to keep pace with the variable state of the patient's mind.

To those sufferers who bask in the sunshine of fortune, and have brought this disease on themselves by allowing their minds to debilitate for want of exertion, how easy to repair the breach, if they would but be guided by the judgment of a friend in the choice of some scientific amusement! When we view the pleasing, the instructive studies of chemistry, mineralogy, botany, &c. and have the pecuniary means of improving our minds in either of those sciences, and making experiments or collections for our own edification, the restoration of our health, and for the benefit of society at large; who that suffers under this distressing malady would not exchange a life of misery for one full of hope, ardour, and expectation? To whom is the world to look for the advancement of science and the arts, if not to the rich? Do not the agriculturists and the country in general benefit by the expensive theories of the opulent landowner? Do not the farmer and the country benefit by the chemical experiments on manure? Is not science aided by geological studies and mineralogical collections? Who but the wealthy can enrich our hot-houses with exotics from foreign countries, in many cases for the advancement of medical science? And who is there that is rich, and has the power of a metamorphosis from languor, debility, and despondency, to energy, strength, and health, that would not make the happy exchange, and who by merely amusing his mind, and enjoying properly the favours of fortune, might leave behind him a name in the cause of science as eminent as that of a Hunter, a Bedford, or a Banks?

What other pursuits will afford the same delights, both mental and bodily? None. In short, employment was designed for us all; and those who are not obliged to labour for their daily bread are bound by every law, human and divine, to spend their fortune, to the utmost of their means, for the attainment of those objects in scientific knowledge, which can only be acquired through the medium of the rich. That such was intended to be the basis of society there can be no doubt; and the Chinese, whom we laugh at, are so convinced of the necessity of employment, that the greatest Mandarin in the state is brought up to some handicraft occupation. It is from not using the gifts of fortune as they were originally designed, that many patients labour under hypochondriasis; for by a little exertion and employment this hydra might be exterminated, and health and spirits reign in its stead.

We shall conclude this long digression by observing, that the want of tone, both of body and mind, will be greatly relieved by the use of the waters, which, strengthening the stomach, and promoting a more healthy action of the secretions, joined with regular exercise, and any occupation calculated to divest the mind of its *ennui*, cannot fail of restoring health to the patient, and rendering him again an useful member of society.

Pyrosis, *or Water-Brash.*

This disorder may likewise be considered a species of dyspepsia. It consists in the discharge of a thin watery fluid from the stomach, sometimes very acrid, but often wholly tasteless, accompanied by a sense of burning heat and pain about the epigastric region. It principally occurs when the stomach is empty, and is supposed to arise from a spasmodic affection of that organ.

Its causes are—violent emotions of the mind, and wet feet, more rarely from organic affection of the stomach. The cases, however, which have come under my observation have evidently arisen from indigestion, and have principally been relieved by the same medicines.

Magnesia and the carbonates of soda and potash are the remedies which give the most immediate relief; still this can only be considered palliative and we must look to some more efficient means for its complete removal. Antispasmodics are likewise advised as an immediate resource, and tonics to strengthen the stomach with occasional purgatives. The *oxyd of bismuth*; *nux nomica*, and various other remedies, have been recommended as specifics; but experience has not justified their claims. The use of opiates, although too often resorted to, we conceive highly prejudicial; the relief they afford being only temporary, but the injury permanent.

This appears to be one of those stomach complaints which, upon every principle, come within the beneficial range of the Bath waters. It is seldom accompanied with much fever, is very frequently of long standing, and attended with many of the visceral derangements which occur in dyspepsia. It is, therefore, highly necessary that some active opening medicine should be taken previous to beginning the waters, and even during their use once or twice in the week.

The waters may be taken and increased as they appear to agree; and the bathing at 96° regularly pursued three or four times in the week, as in cases of indigestion, will promote a more active circulation, and produce a determination to the skin, which are both most essential points in this malady. It is also proper to observe the same directions respecting exercise, food, and amusement for the mind.

Having pointed out how decidedly beneficial the exhibition of the Bath waters is considered in all disorders connected with the stomach, we shall now proceed to that class of diseases which most commonly originate in those deranged functions; we allude to hepatic complaints, or affections of the liver.

ON BILIARY AFFECTIONS.

Having alluded in the last chapter to diseases of the liver as a frequent consequence of the irregularities which so often produce dyspepsia, or indigestion, we shall now refer to those manifold bilious affections which pervade so large a class of the community, and which by many eminent physicians are considered to be the foundation of various anomalous cases, hitherto attributed to nerves, &c.

We shall premise, that as hepatitis, or actual inflammation of the liver, does not come within the range of our views, we shall briefly allude to its chronic stage, and those varieties of obstructions, in which, under the thermal treatment, we may look forward with a prospect of success.

Under this head may be considered schirrus, or disease of the liver; deranged functions from torpid action of the liver; or jaundice, whether arising from viscid vitiated bile, or from biliary calculi obstructing the ducts.

SCHIRRUS,

Or actual disease of the liver, generally commences with all the symptoms of dyspepsia, accompanied by a dull obtuse pain about the region of the liver, extending towards the right shoulder. There is, likewise, considerable fulness and enlargement about the liver, attended with restlessness, emaciation, and great depression of spirits. The bowels are inactive, and the secretions unnatural. In the advancement of this disease, when the remedies have not been effectual in arresting its progress, hectic comes on, which usually terminates in pulmonary affection or dropsical affusion.

Persons who have long resided in tropical climates are particularly subject to this disease, and have generally suffered very much from its inflammatory stage prior to their arrival in this country; it is likewise the effect of a worn-out constitution, and may be traced to habits of intemperance and hard drinking. It will, notwithstanding, in many subjects remain for years without much amendment, or even becoming materially worse.

This latter stage of diseased liver is considered the worst, and least likely to receive much permanent benefit from any remedy; where, however, the expectation of cure is not very sanguine, every palliative means will be looked to with anxious hope; and certainly under very discouraging circumstances, the use of the Bath waters has been attended with considerable relief.

To those especially who come from the continent of India, and are particularly subject to bilious affections and chronic disease of the liver, the Bath waters will prove very congenial. In many cases, however, a course of the Cheltenham waters for a few months prior to coming to Bath will prove of great assistance in carrying off the redundancy of vitiated bile, which is most commonly generated in a warm climate. After this preparatory cleansing, the internal use of the Bath waters will promote an appetite, strengthen the tone of the stomach, improve the digestion, and by their friendly warmth every way assist the circulation, as well as correct the secretions. The bathing, likewise, appears to abate the pain, soften the swelling of the liver, and promote a more regular secretion of bile.

In cases of induration, which are most commonly of an aggravated nature, other remedies must likewise be persevered in to assist the above plan. Those principally advised are of the mercurial kind, in combination with such medicines as circumstances may suggest. The greatest attention must also be paid to diet, which should be very light and nourishing; and moderate exercise, as the patient can bear it. All fatigue should be avoided, for the vital spark must be fanned, not forced. So with society; the hypochondriasis attendant on this disorder must be soothed by pleasant society, and the patient as much as possible withdrawn from himself; but even the society of friends should not be too long continued, and should never be boisterous. The spirits over exerted are only proportionably relaxed afterwards.

It must, however, be allowed, that if this schirrous affection be far advanced, or attended with any degree of fever, the waters must not be persevered in; for under such circumstances they will rather aggravate than relieve the disease.

If, likewise, in advanced age there should be such an enlargement of the gland as to produce jaundice by pressure on the biliary ducts, our hopes of ultimate cure are very limited; but the warm bath, even in this hopeless stage, is attended with no bad consequences, but affords a degree of ease to the patient very soothing and consolatory.

It is almost superfluous to add, that when this stage of disease has been induced by irregularities, or hard drinking, nothing but a correct, regular life can give any remedy the smallest chance of success. Not that we are advocates for running into the opposite extreme, where the stomach has been habitually accustomed to the most stimulating liquors. This may be done with less impunity in the earlier stages of hepatic disease; but where there is indurated liver in advanced life from long continued intemperance, a state of collapse would ensue, and dropsy most certainly be the consequence of withdrawing every stimulus from the stomach and constitution. Under such circumstances a little brandy and water may be allowed with advantage, but always under controul.

We shall now consider the other affections which arise either from a redundancy or deficiency of bile, reserving any general remarks to the latter part of this subject. As all irregular actions of the biliary secretions have a tendency to produce jaundice, we shall point out the diagnosis of this disease, and its various modifications.

JAUNDICE

Consists in a yellow colour of the skin over the whole body, and particularly of the *adnata* of the eyes; sometimes accompanied by fever, but very often without any inflammatory disposition.

Independent of the yellowness of the skin and the eyes, this disorder manifests itself by heaviness, lassitude, pain and oppression about the precordia, sickness, costiveness, with a whiteness of the *fæces alvinæ*, and high-coloured water.

It attacks all ages, and is of longer or shorter duration, according to the constitution of the patient, and the nature of the exciting cause.

Its immediate cause may be traced to biliary calculi obstructing the passage of the bile into the duodenum, which forces it into the mass of blood, where, by its circulation, it gives yellowness to the skin, and constitutes jaundice. It may, however, arise from other causes besides gall-stones. Spasmodic stricture of the ducts will produce the same effect; likewise schirri of the liver, by obstructing the passage of the bile, as stated when treating on schirrus. There have, also, been instances of violent emotions of the mind suddenly producing jaundice, without any appearance of calculi; this, however, can only be accounted for on the principle of spasmodic constriction. The remote cause of jaundice may arise from long residence in a warm climate, sedentary occupations, indolence, &c. which promote a redundancy of bile, and favour biliary obstructions.

The cure of jaundice must be accomplished by the removal of the obstructed bile, and by alleviating the immediate painful symptoms; and the recurrence of the disease prevented by avoiding those excitements which originally predisposed to the disorder.

When we consider the various offices which the bile performs in the animal œconomy, it will not be at all wonderful that a derangement of its functions should affect and disorder the whole machine. With regard to the constitution, it may be considered the grand key-stone of the arch, whose structure cannot be perfect whilst this essential is deficient. By mixing with the food in the duodenum it assists digestion, acts as a stimulus to the intestinal canal, and by increasing the peristaltic motion favours the expulsion of the fæces. That such is the fact is demonstrable from the torpor and want of activity in the bowels, which is one of the most troublesome symptoms in deficiency of bile; this secretion being not only requisite for the proper assimilation of the food in the first instance, but equally necessary for the purposes of health through the whole alimentary canal.

The Bath waters from the earliest periods have been strongly recommended in most chronic diseases of the liver; it must, however, be evident that their exhibition is much more favourable in some stages of hepatic disease than others, and we shall endeavour to point out under what circumstances they may be resorted to with confidence.

We must, however, premise, that in all biliary affections these waters can only be considered as a very powerful auxiliary. The aid of medicine, particularly of the mercurial kind, must be administered to remove the obstruction, and relieve that morbid secretion of bile, which in the first case constitutes the jaundice, and in the second the torpor, which, producing vitiated redundancy, lays the foundation of jaundice.

In cases of jaundice arising from schirrus not much benefit can be expected; and where there is the slightest disposition to inflammation, the waters do harm.

Biliary calculi obstructing the cystic duct is one of the most common causes of jaundice, and it is frequently a considerable time before it will pass into the duodenum, or, as is sometimes the case, fall back again into the gall bladder. During the period of the obstruction, the pain felt about the pit of the stomach, and passing towards the back, is extremely violent, and the largest doses of opium have been given without effect. The sickness occasioned by the pain is likewise very distressing; when, however, the calculus passes or retrogrades, the pain and vomiting immediately cease.

The principal object under the above distressing feelings must be to assist in extending this duct, and promoting the passage of the gall-stone; and nothing more effectually contributes to this purpose than immersion in the warm bath, which acts as an external fomentation, and relaxes the contraction. The time of remaining in the bath should be as long as the patient's strength will allow, and the heat at 100°; the increase of heat and length of stay in the bath, if it bring on exhaustion, or even syncope, will relax the duct, and materially assist in the expulsion of the calculus; gentle friction about the seat of the pain should likewise be used whilst in the bath. The pumping should not be advised under the above circumstances; and drinking the water is out of the question, as other means are obliged to be employed for the purpose of relieving the violent pains, and keeping up the action of the bowels.

Upon the same principle the use of the hot bath is particularly serviceable in abating the pain and relaxing the spasmodic constriction of the duct, which we have stated as another cause of jaundice.

Although the internal use of the waters cannot be advised whilst the absolute obstruction exists, yet when once that is removed, they may be taken with the greatest advantage. Their regular use will assist in improving the digestion, and stimulating the liver to perform its proper functions.

Jaundice will likewise arise from torpor of the liver producing a sluggish secretion of the bile, and from its viscid state obstructing the canal. This is a more common cause of jaundice than even from calculi, and may be distinguished from the latter by its coming on without much pain, though it is generally attended with great languor and debility, and is often accompanied with chlorosis.

In this species of jaundice, where the bowels are properly attended to, both the drinking the waters and bathing will be very beneficial. The first by improving the appetite, assisting digestion, and stimulating the languid circulation; and the latter by attenuating the thickened bile, and promoting its regular passage through the biliary ducts.

This latter form of biliary torpor may exist in a considerable degree without producing actual jaundice, although it may be suspected from the sallowness of countenance, languor, debility, great depression of spirits, bad digestion, and irregular action of the bowels. The state of the secretions will, on inspection, shew a very vitiated state of the bile; and if properly attended to, more serious consequences may be prevented.

It is this state of the biliary secretions which gives rise to such a variety of indescribable complaints, which are attributed to a thousand causes rather than the right one; for how can the wheels of the machine move in proper rotation, when the stimulating power which sets them in motion is defective?

But it is not sufficient, even when the morbid state of the secretions is discovered, merely to give opening medicines to carry off the vitiated bile; this is only attempting the cure by halves, and the patient wonders he never gets cured, when he is continually relieving the system of the foul secretions. The fact is, that whilst proper medicine should be directed to carry off what is improper in the liver, or the bowels, some tonic plan should be likewise pursued to strengthen the stomach, stimulate the circulation, and *prevent* the recurrence of improper biliary accumulations. Here it is that the benefit of the Bath waters is decidedly conspicuous; their internal exhibition acts as a gentle tonic, a warm stimulant, an improver of the blood and juices, and a restorer of that equilibrium which should always subsist between the stomach and the liver, and without which harmony disease must ensue. The use of the warm bath will likewise assist in all the above intentions; and, with proper use of medicine in the early stages of this complaint, will stand every chance of being successful.

We do not mean to signify that most cases of jaundice or obstructed bile may not be recovered by the usual remedies without the application of the Bath waters; if such were the case, there would be great mortality throughout the kingdom; but we mean most decidedly to state, that their proper application will shorten the duration of the attack, very considerably mitigate all the painful and distressing symptoms, and what is equally essential, renovate the constitution, and prevent the recurrence of the tendency to the secretion of vitiated bile.

Dr. Lucas observes, "whatever disorders, then, "derive their origin from an acrimony, not acescency, "of the juices; whatever disorders spring from "an alkalescency of the humours, such as a redun-"dance or preternatural acrimony of the bile, with "putrescency in the fluids or bowels; there the "feverish commotions being previously allayed, "Bath waters will be found a sovereign remedy."

"Whenever," says Dr. Oliver, "the gall ducts "are obstructed by colic pains which arise from "spasm, and the bile is by that means thrown back "into the blood, it immediately tinges the lymph, "and changes the whites of the eyes and all the "surface of the skin into a bright lemon colour. "After proper evacuations, the Bath waters are "almost a certain remedy; abating the pains by "their softening, relaxing, and anodyne quality; "and diluting, correcting, and washing away the "acrid particles from the intestines, which brought "on the spasms that stopped the biliary ducts, "and created the disease."

In alluding to biliary calculi, Dr. Falconer observes, "for these the Bath waters are of the "greatest service; and I believe more gall stones "have been observed to be voided during a course "of the Bath waters, than from any other known "medicine."

Sir George Gibbes on Liver Complaints has the following observations: "as excess in the use of "vinous spirit produces that disorder in the sto-"mach, a consequence of which is the liver com-

"plaint now under consideration; and as a well "directed course of Bath water is found eminently "serviceable in this complaint of the stomach; so "do we find that that state of constitution which is "necessary to the production of this disease is "removed by a course of the Bath waters."

Thus from the concurrent testimony of every writer, from Jones and Guidot to the present day, they all agree in the beneficial effects of warm bathing, in cases of derangement of the biliary secretions, whether arising from redundancy or deficiency of bile.

Dr. Saunders observes, "that there is much "sympathy between the brain and the liver, and "that in maniacal persons there is generally a "defect in the secretion of the bile." Violent passions, which can only be considered as modifications of mania, will very much alter the secretion of bile; and all the medical means on earth will not cure a bilious subject, if his passions be not under the controul of his judgment. Thus, when an angry man vents his choler, he is said to dip his pen in gall; which literally means, that all his vitiated bile is stirred up by the demon raging within.

Exercise is absolutely necessary for the removal of bilious obstructions; and a hard-trotting horse, or carriage without springs, may be considered no bad remedy for an incipient jaundice. It is not, however, the mere removal of disease which should be particularly regarded; the various means enumerated above will, with proper perseverance, be sure to accomplish this end, if the disease be not organic, or a preliminary to ascites. It is the prevention of its recurrence which should be the grand desideratum, and this can only be effected in two ways—the first by avoiding those causes which tend to the disease; the second, by pursuing the restorative means which the Bath waters are so well calculated to accomplish. The exciting causes in many hepatic diseases are similar to those enumerated under the heads of indigestion and hypochondriasis; and it must be very evident, in attending to the history of the above disorders, and those of which we are now treating, that they are modifications of the same disease, or, we should rather say, different stages of their progress, that the same precautions are necessary in avoiding stimulating and improper food, which weakens the powers of digestion; that the same exercise and attention to the bowels are to be observed for the prevention of improper accumulations; and that the same intellectual means should be pursued to expel that torpor which exists in all the functions —the stomach, the liver, and the brain. To the above regulations we must strenuously advise the steady use of the Bath waters, both as regards the bathing and the drinking. Their intentions have been already stated; and well convinced are we by long experience, that those who will, under proper management, confide in their good effects, will not be disappointed in their expectations.

The disease of jaundice, of course, has never been considered infectious; yet a remarkable instance occurred in the family of Capt. Fitzgerald, R. N. where four of the children, the youngest about four years old, were one after the other, in regular succession, seized with jaundice. Although there was some degree of languor and want of their usual spirits in these youthful subjects, yet the complaint was unattended by any feverish symptoms, pains, or, indeed, hardly any indisposition, and was soon relieved by a little mercurial medicine. At first I conceived it probable that the obstruction might occur from the milk diet; but if that were possible, why did it not produce the disease earlier? the same food constituting their nourishment both before and since. No other cause could be discovered.

Mr. K., a young gentleman of fortune, whilst pursuing a round of amusements in this fashionable city, was seized with a violent pain in his bowels, (as he expressed it,) considerable nausea, and great costiveness. His countenance was very sallow; and on examination of the fæces, I discovered a total suppression of bile. In a few days the colour of the skin changed almost to a black jaundice; his bowels, although relieved with difficulty by pretty active mercurial medicine, still shewed that the biliary obstruction was not removed, and the other secretions were equally indicative of the disease. The pain between the stomach and bowels had subsided to a dull obtuse feel, and there was not the slightest degree of fever. For ten days the medicines were persevered in without removing the obstruction; he then went into a warm bath at 98°, and continued in half an hour; the next day he bathed again; and after the third bathing the appearances were changed, and the pain had entirely subsided. By a continuance of the bathing, and occasional doses of mercury, in three weeks he left Bath perfectly well of the disease, and the skin gradually recovering its natural appearance.

Dr. Baynard gives the following evidence of the benefit of the Bath waters in affections of the liver.

Mr. H., of an ill habit from an irregular life, came to Bath: he complained in the right hypochondria and region of the liver, and had a great induration there; yet this man, by drinking, purging, and bathing, got a perfect cure.

Mrs. T. received a great cure by the Bath waters, joined with some other operatives, in as high a jaundice as ever was seen, which had long seized her, and she a very lean, emaciated, worn out woman. And in this case, and also most diseases of the liver, I think the

Bath waters the best specific in the world, if taken seasonably, with due preparatives and advice, &c. &c.

Mrs. E. laboured under a constant vomiting, with racking pain about the orifice of the stomach. She had neither retained food nor medicine for a month. Supposing her complaints owing to biliary concretions then passing the duct, I told her this was truly a Bath case. With great difficulty she was transported to Bath. When I first saw her, her pains were exquisite; she threw up laudanum, and every other thing. She was lodged in one of those houses from whence there is a slip or communication into the bath. I advised her to drink a glass of water at any time in bed, and as fast as she threw that up another; and so continue till she was sure the water began to stay on her stomach. She was also carried into the bath, sometimes twice in a morning, and there supported till she began to vomit. While she was in the bath her pains ceased. In a few days the water began to stay. At once she passed twenty-two gall-stones, as big as beans and peas, by stool: at different times more. Her pain vanished. From a skeleton (in less than three weeks) she grew plump, and walked on the Parade.

She went home. Her complaints returned. She came again to Bath, where she pursued the same regimen, and found her cure. Profiting by experience she staid six months; during which time she drank about a quart of water a day, and swallowed two pounds and upwards of soap every week. For eight years past she has enjoyed perfect health, excepting grumbling remembrances of her pain, which she continues to lull by the constant use of soap, and Bath water warmed at home.

M. H., aged 66 years, for a length of time subject to the gout. Fifteen years ago, in one of these fits, he turned yellow, and took medicines for the jaundice. In April last he was seized with a violent pain in his stomach, which pain he was subject to by fits; but was now more than ordinary fainty, the jaundice appearing presently in his water, but not in his eyes, face, and skin, till about a month after. By the advice of Radcliff and others he took medicines to little purpose. He came to Bath the last day of August, so weak and ill, that he could hardly keep life in him. The night after he had a most violent colic fit, in which he strained very much to vomit. He was yellow all over. He set presently about drinking the waters, (being in continual pain, and stomachless,) but at first in small quantities. The third time of taking them he voided a gall-stone about the bigness of a pigeon's egg, with several lesser pieces of the same colour and consistence, a *sabulum* to the quantity of a spoonful and more. It is observable, that this gentleman had a stool before the stone came off, as white and like to tobacco-pipe clay; but the stool that came with and after the stone was as yellow as saffron. He was immediately more at ease; he recovered by degrees; he goes on drinking the waters, this being the one and twentieth day of his cure; walks abroad, pays visits, eats heartily, and is very likely to recover perfectly.

Mr. D. came hither in February, in the 60th year of his age. His complaints were (beside the yellowness of of his skin) weakness, faintness, decay of spirits, shaking in his hands, pain in his limbs, doughy swellings of the legs, clamminess of his mouth, drought, and foulness of the tongue. He had but lately undergone purging, and therefore had the less need of preparation. He took at first but two pints, then three, then two quarts, seldom exceeding. They passed freely by stool and urine. Between whiles he was, however, purged with rhubarb and calomel; he took alteratives, and now and then intermitted the waters. About the middle of his course he was let blood, which had a quantity of serum tinctured yellow. About the latter end of his course he bathed three or four times; he had before bathed his legs and feet to get down the swelling, which answered. He apparently got vigour and strength, a clearer countenance, and better habit of body. Thus he returned after two months' stay. He came to Bath again in May, and staid about the same time with manifest advantage.

The next is a case of Dr. Pierce's, where, contrary to our present mode of directing the waters, bathing was not recommended; still the cure was effected by improving the stomach and clearing the passages.

The Rev. Mr. B. came down very weak, faint, and stomachless, about the middle of April. His chief complaints were decay of spirits and strength, chiefly in his back. The remedies he had taken he thought took off his stomach, for he could digest nothing; all things that he ate came up again; he was withal in great pain, so that he could not sleep at night, nor was he at ease by day, in any posture, whether sitting, walking, standing, or lying. At length the jaundice appeared, by the yellowness of his skin and the whites of his eyes. Under these weak circumstances he came hither, and was so faint and enfeebled, that he contented himself with a small chamber, not being able to go up stairs to a larger and better room. I put him upon drinking these waters, bathing not being at all likely to agree with him; nor did he, as I remember, once bathe at all. It was more than a week or ten days before he could discover the least alteration for the better; but at length the water passing well opened his body, (which was apt to be costive before,) cleared the passages, restored his stomach, and abated his pains, by which he was enabled to sleep, eat, and digest, (and consequently to get strength, which he did in every part but his back, where some weakness, more or less, hath still continued.) He came a second time the same year, about August, and was then so much amended, that he that could be hardly heard to speak in a wide chamber, (his lungs and voice were so weak when he came first,) before he went away preached in our large church with great applause.

ON UTERINE DISEASES.

We shall now consider those maladies which are peculiar to the female sex; and still adhering to the original design of giving a slight account of each disorder, shall, with as much delicacy and brevity as possible, point out those uterine affections which may claim the assistance of these celebrated springs.

Under this class of diseases we shall omit the insertion of cases, and have no doubt the motive will be readily perceived. The utility of the Bath waters, however, in these complaints has been so long and generally acknowledged, as to make this omission of no material consequence.

Although modern authors in general have been very reluctant in allowing the benefit of warm bathing in other diseases, yet in all those uterine affections which have come under consideration, its beneficial effects have been too apparent to withstand their recommendation. And with the greatest justice it may be observed, that no remedy exists, so safe, so pleasant, or so effectual, as the Bath waters, in giving strength to the stomach, action to the liver, and tone to the debility of the uterine vessels. For it is a combination of all these affections which constitutes the class of diseases under our present notice.

Chlorosis, *or Retention of the Catamenia.*

This disorder, known under the appellation of chlorosis, or green sickness, attacks young women about the age of thirteen, or at that period when regular menstruation should appear; indeed, it is the deficiency in this respect which constitutes the malady. As menstruation, however, commences at all periods between the ages of twelve and eighteen, or even twenty years, the want of such a flow at the usual time is not to be considered as disease, unless accompanied by those unequivocal deviations from health we are about to enumerate.

The usual symptoms of chlorosis are, great debility, loss of appetite, or one very depraved, indolence, lassitude, fatigue, and great shortness of breath on the slightest exertion, pallid face, violent palpitation of the heart, swollen and tense bowels, together with a train of hysterical and dyspeptic symptoms.

These are generally accompanied by a great disposition to costiveness; whilst distressing pains are felt about the back, loins, and lower limbs, the latter being very subject to œdematous swellings. There exists at the same time great coldness of the extremities, and a general want of circulation.

These symptoms constitute chlorosis, and hardly ever appear separate from a retention of the menses.

The cause of this disease is generally acknowledged to depend entirely on weakness and a want of power to propel the blood with sufficient energy into the uterine vessels. It frequently proves one of a very formidable nature; and if not relieved, terminates fatally, either by inducing pulmonary affections, or a diseased state of the viscera.

The stomach is always considerably disordered, and the powers of digestion much impaired; indeed it has been suggested, that chlorosis has its origin in a deranged state of the stomach and bowels, and that by active treatment of the bowels alone the disease is effectually removed.

As far as my observation goes, the very reverse appears to be the case; the diseased state of the stomach, and torpid action of the liver and bowels, are merely symptomatic of the state of the uterine vessels; and when by the assistance of warm bathing and tonic medicines a more general circulation is promoted, and the action of the uterus restored, the dyspeptic symptoms immediately disappear, the appetite returns, the palpitations cease, the colour reappears in the cheeks, and the bowels perform their functions without the aid of those drastic purgatives, which, under other circumstances, would almost destroy the suffering patient.

Dr. Hamilton,* to whom we alluded in the foregoing observations, denies chlorosis to be caused by retention or suppression of the catamenia. He asserts the disease to arise from costiveness, and endeavours to prove that perseverance in purgative medicines will cure the complaint. His own words we shall quote.

" Impressed with these considerations, and with " a previous favourable opinion of the utility of " purgative medicines in other complaints, I " many years ago adopted the use of them in " chlorosis. I expected, by obviating costiveness, " to remove the stomachic symptoms, and of course " others that depended upon them. I pursued this " practice with the greater readiness, because I had " experienced, on many occasions, the uncertain " and protracted cure of chlorosis by the remedies " in common use. Scarcely had I begun the " exhibition of purgative medicines in chlorosis,

* Hamilton on Purgatives, p. 61.

"when I had the satisfaction to find that the "opinion which I had formed of them was well "founded, and that they proved at once safe and "quickly salutary."

In proof of the above theory Dr. Hamilton asserts, that young men are subject to chlorosis as well as females. Alluding, likewise, to Dr. Cullen's opinion, that this disease arises from defective circulation of the uterine vessels, he observes, "but opposed to this theory a still more con-"clusive argument is drawn from the circumstance "of chlorosis appearing occasionally among the "more feeble and delicate of the male sex; for "although females are attacked more frequently "and more severely with chlorosis, yet it is not "peculiar to them."

Never having met with any of these chlorotic young gentlemen, it is needless to enter into a discussion on that point. One observation may be made with regard to the Doctor's hypothesis; —if costiveness produce chlorosis, why does not the latter disease occur at every period of life, or connected with other disorders? or why should the accession of the catamenia invariably cure the disease, and all the unpleasant symptoms connected with it?

But to prove more strongly that Dr. Hamilton has mistaken the effect for the cause, we need only deduce those cases of chlorosis which arise from sudden suppression, from any violent excitement, or exposure to damp. In such cases the derangement of the system is immediately accompanied by pallid looks, tense body, very confined bowels, depraved appetite, &c.; and these symptoms will certainly continue till the uterine obstruction be removed.

It will not be denied that the use of purgatives assists very decidedly in the removal of this complaint, and indeed in the removal of most other disorders which "flesh is heir to;" and every author who has treated on the subject of chlorosis has recommended stimulating the rectum by active purgatives, with a view of exciting the action of the uterine vessels. The medical world are very much indebted to Dr. Hamilton for drawing their attention more decidedly to the beneficial effects of purgatives; but the above observations only shew to what extent a favourite theory may be carried.

The principal remedies usually recommended by authors for the removal of this distressing malady, (which unfortunately proves the *grave* of thousands,) are tonics and cold bathing, with occasional active purgatives. The mind kept at ease, with moderate exercise, either walking or on horseback, have also been considered, and most properly, powerful auxiliaries.

I have been more particular in entering into a general statement of this disease, because I am convinced, there is no malady so certainly and so effectually relieved as this is by the assistance of the Bath waters; but before I state the benefit derived from the hot bathing, I shall take a cursory view of the use of the cold bath, and give Dr. Reid's able observations on the cold treatment in this particular disease.

Dr. Reid,* who had many years practical knowledge of the good and bad effects of warm and cold sea bathing, has given a very able chapter on the subject of chlorosis. After stating his opinion of the nature of the disease, which coincides with that of Dr. Cullen and others, as arising from a debility of the uterine vessels, he draws the following conclusion:

"There is no complaint in which cold bathing "is so universally recommended, as in every stage "of chlorosis, and very often with the wished-for "success; change of air and moderate exercise "being peculiarly well adapted to such cases. But "before it is attempted, the caution so often re-"peated must be carefully observed; whether a "sufficient degree of energy is present in the sys-"tem to bear the shock of the water, and produce "the reaction and succeeding warm sensation. "Of the many chlorotic cases that have come

* Reid on Warm and Cold Sea Bathing, p. 59.

"under my notice of late years, it may be with "truth affirmed, that *scarcely half of them have* "*been relieved by cold bathing*, even when con- "tinued a considerable time. When the strength "is much reduced, the countenance pale and "bloated, the lower limbs œdematous, retaining "the impression, bathing in the sea is not advise- "able, for the reasons already given when treating "of general debility."

So much for the cold bathing; and from the Doctor's experience of its bad success, he gives his *amended treatment*, which consists in clearing out the stomach and bowels, and advising a warm sea bath every night, or three times in the week, remaining in it as long as the patient can bear, or beginning with five minutes, and gradually prolonging the time to half an hour, and during the immersion to apply gentle friction to the lower limbs. To this plan may be added such tonics as are suitable, with moderate exercise, cheerful company, and amusements that are not fatiguing.

By the above candid statement Dr. Reid acknowledges that *not one half* of his chlorotic patients were relieved by the cold bathing; but that on failure, and trying the warm bath, he relates instances of complete success.

Dr. Saunders* likewise gives his testimony in favour of the Bath waters in the following words:

* Saunders on Mineral Waters, p. 184.

"Chlorosis (a disease which is at all times much "relieved by steel, and will bear it, even where "there is considerable degree of feverish irritation) "is often entirely removed by a course of Bath "water; and its use as a warm bath will greatly "contribute to remove that languor of circulation, "and obstruction of the natural evacuations, which "constitute the leading features of this troublesome "disorder."

Dr. Falconer observes, "in that species of chlo-"rosis which is attended with paleness, diminution "of strength, and depraved appetite, the Bath "waters are generally successful, and may be used "in all cases where chalybeate medicines are "proper."*

The truth is, that in no class of diseases are the Bath waters more efficacious, or more to be relied on, than in obstinate cases of chlorosis. Their internal and external use in all retentions and suppressions has been long and deservedly recommended; and in a period of twenty years I have never seen a case (unconnected with organic disease) that was not ultimately relieved, if properly persevered in.

It is, perhaps, impossible to lay down a general rule of procedure with regard to the Bath waters for the various patients who may apply for relief labouring under this disorder. This must of

* Falconer on the Bath Waters, p. 339.

course be regulated by the medical attendant according to the stage of the disease and the state of the patient. It is, however, usual, after cleansing the *primæ viæ*, to begin the waters in small quantities at the weakest pump, gradually increasing as the stomach is able to bear them ; bathing, likewise, from 96 to 98 degrees of heat, two or three times in the week, and remaining in the bath from ten to thirty or forty minutes, according to the strength of the patient; gentle friction whilst in the bath : and in addition to these means, the greatest benefit arises from pumping on the loins to the amount of two or three hundred strokes, either in the bath, or on the alternate days of bathing, if the patient's strength will admit of the dry pump.

As the principal means of removing chlorosis consists in exciting the action of the vessels of the uterus, and propelling the blood into them more copiously, it is easy to conceive how the warm bathing and pumping act mechanically in assisting this determination. They likewise promote a more general and regular circulation through the whole of the capillary vessels, which in this disease are all equally obstructed. Thus the bathing and pumping, by mechanically stimulating the vessels, are most materially assisted by the internal use of the waters, and other strengthening medicines, which, according to the urgency and violence of the case, may be requisite.

Many cases of retention are relieved after a short use of the Bath waters; but it must be evident that obstinate cases, attended with great debility, and of long standing, require regular and steady perseverance. It is often advisable, after the trial of a month or six weeks, to leave them off for a fortnight, and then begin again; this, however, must be left to the discretion of the medical attendant. Dr. Charlton, in his enumeration of cases, mentions several patients, who, after three months' steady perseverance in bathing, pumping, and drinking, received little or no benefit, yet eventually were entirely cured by the waters; and this fact cannot be too strongly impressed on the mind of the patient, that the benefit of the waters is not always felt immediately on their application, and frequently not until their use has been discontinued; but that in those diseases where their exhibition is proper, particularly in uterine affections, their action, though slow, is nevertheless sure.

Suppression of the Catamenia.

Any interruption to the flow of the catamenia, after it has once been regularly established, is considered a suppression.

The symptoms of this disease in many respects resemble those of retention, being attended with severe pains in the head, back, and loins, with hysteric and dyspeptic symptoms, great costiveness, and violent colic pains.

Our opinion of this disease and its consequences is formed from a knowledge of its cause, suppression being seldom or never an idiopathic disease, though considered such by many writers.

If suppression have taken place from exposure to cold, violent emotion, or any sudden cause, the blood is often diverted from the uterus to some other part, and occasions hemorrhagies. Suppression will sometimes occur from general debility of the system ; it is also in many instances the effect of other diseases ; such is the fact in pulmonary and paralytic affections, and in those cases it can only be cured by a removal of the cause.

Although cold bathing has been so generally recommended in retention, yet in this disease Dr. Cullen, and other authors copying from him, has advised the warm bath, together with antispasmodics and general stimulants. Our opinion of the superior efficacy of the warm bath in retention has been already stated ; and in this complaint the removal of the constriction of the uterine vessels being the grand desideratum, the warm bath, aided by friction and pumping on the loins, and the chalybeate and stimulating property of the

Bath waters taken internally, seldom fail in soon effecting relief. "*A purgationibus reficiendæ sunt* "*mulieres diebus paucis insequutis; exercendæ* "*ambulationibus, inferiorum frictionibus, et bal-* "*neo.*" *Paulus Ægineta de mensium suppressione.*

All the class of diseases connected with the uterus are more decidedly benefited by the Bath waters than by any known remedy; and many instances are recorded, where every means had been tried without effect for removing retention and suppression prior to the application of these waters.

In certain cases of suppression much caution is necessary previous to the use of the waters, and recourse should not be had to them unadvisedly. I allude particularly to those cases which occur suddenly from any violent cause, and occasion great determination of blood to the head. Under these circumstances topical or general bleeding, with active purgatives, must be resorted to, before the the waters can be recommended with safety.

There are a variety of other remedies advised in this complaint; but our great object in these pages is to impress on the mind that the sheet anchor is the Bath waters, and any co-operation they may require must be left to the discretion of the physician.

There is one very essential advantage attending the use of the Bath waters in this disease, which should not be overlooked. A doubt sometimes exists, whether the suppression may not be owing to pregnancy; and medical men are often very cautious in the medicines they administer on that account; and many, not conversant with the peculiar properties of the Bath waters in this respect, might suppose the bathing to be injurious; such, however, is not the case, as warm bathing from the earliest periods has been recommended with the view of assisting delivery and preventing miscarriage. "*Cæterum mense nono relaxandi corporis* "*gratia in pregnantibus, balneo frequenter utendum est; et omni ratione prospiciendum, ut* "*paritura futuros partus dolores fortiter possit* "*ferre.*" *Ætius de Balneis.*

Difficult Menstruation.

The name of this complaint designates the nature of the disease. It is of very common occurrence, and is attended by severe pains in the back, loins, and bottom of the belly. These symptoms come on at the usual return of the catamenia, which appears with difficulty, and in very diminished quantity. It is occasioned either by general debility or spasm in the uterine vessels.

Should debility of constitution be the cause, the same plan should be rigorously pursued as directed for retention and suppression. Under other circumstances the warm bathing, for a few times prior to the accession of the catamenia, has proved of the greatest service, in taking off spasm and removing the constriction of the vessels. In these cases of deficient menstruation the pumping on the loins should never be omitted, provided the patient be able to bear it; and the occasional use of sedatives in relieving the excessive pain materially assists the thermal plan.

With some patients it occurs very slightly, with others it is more painful and distressing; nevertheless its alleviation may be looked upon as most certain by the assistance of the bath, provided it is unconnected with organic disease.

Cessation of Catamenia.

By cessation of catamenia I do not mean obstruction, but that cessation which occurs at the proper period of life, but is attended frequently with distressing flushings, &c.

I am not inclined to think that the Bath waters internally are of much benefit for the indisposition sometimes felt about this period. They are rather too stimulating, and too apt to determine towards the head. With great attention to the bowels, I have seen much benefit by occasional bathing about 92° or 94° in relieving those flushings which frequently arise from irregularity of circulation. Should the patient, however, be of a full habit, topical or general bleeding, with active purgatives, would be prudent, previous to the use of even the warm bath. The pediluvium may always be used with advantage.

MENORRHAGIA, *or Excess of the Catamenia.*

" *Dorsi, lumborum, ventris, parturientium in-* " *star, dolores; menstruorum copiosior, vel san-* " *guinis e vaginâ præter ordinem fluxus.*"*

The excess we are about to describe is not that arising from or connected with child-bearing, but that redundancy which most frequently has its origin in a plethoric habit, and a consequent debility of the uterine vessels.

In the beginning it is often attended by violent head-aches, severe pains about the back, loins, and

* Cullen.

lower limbs, considerable fever, and strong symptoms of hysteria. From a continuation of this complaint, and its frequent repetition, the face becomes pale, the pulse weak, an unusual debility is felt in exercise, the breathing is hurried, pains and coldness are felt in the lower extremities, and a dangerous state of debility is induced.

There are various causes which may produce this complaint. It may arise from general fulness of habit, or be occasioned by severe exercise, violent emotions, general laxity of fibre, or organic disease.

Where this malady arises from organic affection, that is, from ulceration, schirrus, polypus, &c. our hopes of ùltimate cure are very feeble, and the only remedies are those of a palliative nature, such as opium, &c. with local applications. Its occurrence between the ages of forty and fifty would always make us apprehensive of its connexion with organic disease.

Where, however, it occurs at earlier periods of life, and it can be accounted for on the principle of fulness, this disposition must be diverted by bleeding, and avoiding every stimulant and exciting food. Exercise should be avoided, and the patient should observe a light cool diet, and be kept in a horizontal posture.

If, however, instead of plethora, the frequent returns or long continuance of the complaint have produced general debility, emaciated frame, with hysterical and dyspeptic symptoms; it becomes, then, absolutely necessary that some steps should be taken to correct the malady, and renovate the constitution. One certain symptom may always be relied upon; if the disease have continued so long as to be succeeded by leucorrhæa, this of itself points out the necessity of early attention.

Notwithstanding the above, nature should not be inproperly interfered with, for the circumstance of too great a flow occurring at any particular period can only be ascertained by the debilitating effects it may produce. It is frequently the case with young people to be very abundant in this respect, and the flow often recurs at earlier periods than is usual; still if the health be not affected, a redundance should always be preferred to a deficiency, as the latter very often leads to retention.

When all the inflammatory symptoms have been subdued by the usual means, and debility alone remains, the internal use of the Bath waters has proved very efficacious; but in cases of very great weakness their benefit is much assisted by the use of tonic medicines, particularly the different preparations of steel, and the sulphate of zinc.

Great attention must be paid to the bowels, and every exciting cause avoided which can in any way dispose to a return of the disorder; for an early observance of these rules may prevent a train of miseries, the foundation of most organic diseases of the uterus arising from neglect in the first instance.

The greatest benefit has also been derived from local applications; they should not, however, be used in the early stages; the most effectual appears to be a strong solution of alum, or the decoction of oak bark.

Bathing and pumping are sometimes of service, but they should not be recommended as a general rule. In some cases of full sanguine temperament they would be very apt to propel the blood with too great force to the uterine vessels, and bring on the disease we are endeavouring to rectify.

The various modifications of menorrhagia can only be successfully treated by the aid of the Bath waters, under the discerning eye of the professional attendant; for so different is this disease in different individuals, that in one class of patients the most active stimulants might be proper, and in another class the treatment should be diametrically opposite.

We shall now proceed to give a short account of leucorrhæa, which may be considered a disease of local debility, principally arising from long continued menorrhagic affection.

Leucorrhæa, *or Fluor Albus*,

"*Est præternaturalis humoris pituitosi et albi,* "*vel varii coloris et odoris per muliebria excre-* "*tio, orta a nimiâ vasorum uterinorum laxitate et* "*debilitate.*"

This discharge is supposed by Dr. Cullen to proceed from the laxity of the extreme vessels of the uterus. Sydenham apprehends it to arise not only from the vessels of the uterus, but also from the glands of the vagina.

The quantity of discharge varies considerably; but by long continuance it grows more acrid, excoriating the passage, and producing great heat and irritation. Symptoms of general debility supervene, with disordered stomach, and pains about the back and loins.

The causes of this complaint are general and local weakness, and are very similar to those described under the head of menorrhagia; its consequences, in ultimately producing organic disease, are also similar.

It occurs at all ages, from the earliest to the latest period; it is, however, a disease more commonly affecting those in the prime of life, and generally symptomatic.

Of all the disorders to which the female sex are liable, leucorrhæa is the most troublesome and distressing; and the consequences of its neglect are never sufficiently considered, until it lays the foundation of those organic affections, which entail on the unfortunate sufferers a lingering and miserable existence.

Its first advances are often little attended to; and, from its nature and other circumstances, it is suffered to gain ground, when a little timely assistance would at once arrest its progress. It should always be remembered, that in this complaint, likewise, the earlier the application for advice, the more effectual must be the relief; for if suffered to continue any length of time sterility is almost a certain consequence.

The treatment here is both constitutional and local, and very similar to that recommended for menorrhagia; the only difference is, that the Bath water is more decidedly useful in this disease in all its stages, leucorrhæa being invariably a disorder of debility, menorrhagia sometimes quite the contrary, though from long continuance it generally terminates in exhaustion.

In cases of fluor albus Hoffman recommends a course of mineral waters with the greatest confidence; and all our writers on the Bath waters have testified to their surprising effect in this debilitating complaint.

The waters at the King's pump are usually recommended with the greatest advantage; also bathing and pumping on the back and loins, in or out of the bath, as the strength of the patient will allow. The latter remedy wonderfully relieves the heavy, wearing pains about the lumbar region, and gives a tone and energy to the circulation, which is generally very deficient.

In addition to these remedies, the use of stimulating injections must be attended to; the most efficacious and the least objectionable is one ounce of alum dissolved in a pint of rain water, and used cold three times in the day.

With regard to diet much must depend on the state of the patient; in general it should be light and nourishing, and a glass or two of good red wine is often an useful assistant. The bowels should be kept regular, and the quantum of exercise regulated by the strength and ability of the patient. In no two cases can general directions be precisely the same.

What other remedies may be necessary in conjunction with the waters cannot here be decided; but half measures are of little avail in this class of complaints of long standing, and a cure must not be expected without steady perseverance.

Indeed, these diseases are often a considerable time in their progress before they are noticed; and probably, did not the inroads they make on the constitution arrest the attention of the patient's relatives or friends, the disorder might be suffered to go on until all human aid would be ineffectual. Some of the most obstinate of these cases have received the greatest benefit from the united effects of the Bath waters; and where barrenness has long been the consequence, they have not only got rid of the disorder, but have been fortunate in procuring "an heir to their expectations." "*Balneis* "*utantur qui conceptum fieri cupiunt, neque as*-"*siduis neque copiosis.*" *Ætius de Balneis.*

Hysteria.

This disorder we consider to be symptomatic of some derangement of the uterus, and of course affecting *females only*, and those particularly about the menstrual period. It is very similar in many of its symptoms to hypochondriasis; thus what we should term the latter in the male sex, we should consider an hysterical affection in females.

It is very difficult to describe the exact symptoms of an hysteric fit, they occur so differently in different subjects, according to the nature of the exciting cause. Its usual indications are, a convulsive motion about the abdomen, and the sensation of a ball ascending from thence to the stomach and throat, occasioning a feel of suffocation; great distension and flatulence; convulsive motions of the face, limbs, and whole body; alternate fits of laughing and crying, with incoherent talking, &c. These attacks, after subsiding a short time, will often recur, until the patient is quite exhausted, and sinks into a state of stupor or insensibility, from which she awakes unconscious of the circumstances that occurred during the fit. Other symptoms will occasionally be felt, such as head-ache, palpitation of the heart, frequent sighing, and distressing hiccup, with great depression of spirits prior to an attack.

Its causes are, emotions of the mind, or derangement of the functions of the uterus, particularly chlorosis, menorrhagia, or leucorrhæa; and like those maladies, hysteria is frequently accompanied by a disordered state of the digestive organs.

The principal treatment requisite for the cure of this affection is, first, the application of immediate remedies for the removal of the fit; and secondly, an endeavour to obviate the cause, and so brace the constitution as to prevent a recurrence; for hysterical affections are very apt to become habitual, and in that case very difficult to remove.

If the patient be of a full habit, bleeding and antispasmodics are recommended for the relief of the fit; but if the attacks are accompanied by either of the three uterine diseases just stated, the same directions as to the waters and other means will be necessary, for it can, under these circumstances, only be considered as symptomatic.

This disorder is, however, very much under the controul of the patient, where it arises from violent passions, or indulgence in melancholy subjects; and mental exertion will more effectually conquer the complaint than any medicinal means.

As this affection can, with more propriety, only be considered as one of the unpleasant symptoms attending those uterine diseases, of which we have already treated, and as we have so strongly recommended a trial of the Bath waters in those maladies, so we can with equal confidence advise their use as a prevention of hysteria.

Steadily pursuing the drinking, bathing, and pumping, with great attention to the bowels, moderate exercise, and cheerful company, and withal a determination to exert the energies of the mind, cannot fail of effecting a cure in a disorder, which is not more afflicting to the patient than distressing to the friends and attendants.

Chorea Sancti Viti.

St. Vitus's Dance takes its name from St. Vitus's chapel, where in the spring of the year the young people of both sexes used to meet to dance; and dancing in a whimsical and enthusiastical way brought on this convulsive malady;—thus far the fabulous origin of its name.

The disorder itself consists in a convulsive motion of the muscles of different limbs, principally occurring on one side, and affecting young people of both sexes between the ages of 10 and 16 years.

With females this convulsion may often be attributed to hysteria, and connected with a change of life; thus when the latter takes place, the disorder very generally subsides. It does, however, occur after that period, but is often symptomatic of some uterine derangement; and very singular cases have been attested by various authors.

Independent of the above excitements, it may often arise from local irritation, such as worms, teething, local injuries, &c. or it may be occasioned by mental agitation, objects of horror or disgust, &c.

But the most singular character of this malady is, that it sometimes arises from sympathy, and the whole ward of a hospital have been set dancing by the antics of one case of chorea. This in some degree corroborates its history.

It is impossible to enumerate the various ways in which this disorder will shew itself; sometimes by blinking or a convulsed motion of the muscles of the eye; at other times the face is twisted and distorted on one side ; in some cases one arm is suddenly thrown in a direction contrary to the will ; when sitting down, the knees will jump up, or the head be thrown back; in short, every case is different with regard to its form, although its identity is very easily detected.

In most of those cases which have fallen under my observation, it has generally occurred to females between the ages of twelve and sixteen ; but after the latter age, and the settlement of the constitution, the unpleasant symptoms have invariably disappeared.

In the treatment of chorea, tonics and sea bathing have usually been recommended, and in plethoric habits, bleeding and purgatives; from the latter remedy Dr. Hamilton found the greatest benefit, when every other means had failed. The various modes of treatment must, however, be discretionally advised, according to the age and strength of the patient, and the exciting cause of the disease.

Where chorea attacks females, and it appears to be connected with the period of life, after the use of purgatives, the Bath waters may be administered with the greatest advantage. Their internal exhibition will strengthen the stomach without overloading it ; and their external application diffuse a general warmth, particularly in the lower extremities, which is often very deficient. They will likewise promote that accession which is the desirable object.

Dr. Charlton states, that out of eight cases of chorea St. Viti admitted into the General Hospital, three were discharged cured, three much better, and two received no benefit. Dr. Falconer observes, that, out of nine cases admitted for this complaint, eight were cured, and one better. He further remarks, after stating the benefit derived from the Bath waters, " in those cases that I have " seen, bathing and pumping the spine of the back " moderately twice or three times a week seemed " to be the principal circumstances that led towards " the cure."

Where this disease is occasioned by local irritation, from teeth, wounds, &c. nothing but a removal of the cause can afford relief ; and where it arises from a defective state of the digestive functions, the treatment for that class of disorders should be strictly pursued ; it was under these circumstances that Dr. Hamilton's plan proved so efficacious. Electricity is also recommended, but with very doubtful success.

In the year 1812, I was sent for to a young lady, about the age of thirteen, tall and thin, who had been seized with a convulsive motion of the lower limbs, very painful to herself, and distressing to her parents. When seated on a chair or the sofa, she would be suddenly attacked by violent spasmodic twitchings of the muscles of the lower limbs, which would throw her knees towards her chin, and if stooping at all, would strike the chin with great violence. This spasm generally continued for two or three minutes, and then subsided, leaving a dull obtuse pain about the limbs, and considerable languor and debility. The attacks would occur four or five times in the day, and sometimes, though not so frequently, in the night. In other respects her health was good, though the countenance appeared sallow, and the bowels were very confined. Supposing this complaint to arise from some change about to take place, she was directed to take a calomel pill and opening medicine, and the feet to be immersed in Bath water for three nights. This plan seemed to produce some benefit, but not much; she in consequence bathed every other day, with two hundred strokes of the pump upon the loins, and active opening medicine the intermediate days. After a fortnight's perseverance the spasms subsided, and by a continuance of the bathing and pumping for six weeks, a change in the constitution took place, and the patient never had a return of the chorea.

I have met with many slight indications of chorea, and have invariably stopt their progress by using purgatives and the warm bath; and in most cases, if application be made in time, think the disease may be prevented. Strong nervous antispasmodic medicines, with opium, &c. considerably aggravate the disease, and prevent the full efficacy of the depleting system. The two following cases of chorea are related, the first by Dr. Oliver, the other by Dr. Charlton, both being benefited by the Bath waters.

Thomas Neale, aged 13, had been subject to various and strange fits, which the vulgar imputed to witchcraft, (as usually they do whatsoever is not common.) It seemed to me to be a complication of convulsion, epilepsy, and chorea Sancti Viti, and (to be sure) a high scorbute affecting chiefly the brain and the nervosum genus. Out of the fits he would be greatly disordered in his head; sometimes talked at random, sometimes could not speak at all. He had for the most part irregular motions in his arms and hands, legs and feet; tottered so that they could not trust him to ride (scarcely stand) alone. He remained five or six weeks, or more, in which time, by drinking the waters and bathing, and using antiscorbutic, antiepileptic, and chalybeate alteratives, was so recovered as to walk, talk, and carry himself composedly, and to ride home alone; and continued from that time well, without any relapse; and is since (as I hear) become a healthy man, and married.

Mary Ford, of a sanguine and robust constitution, aged 26, was admitted into the Hospital, under my care. Her complaint was an involuntary motion of her right arm. It was occasioned by a fright, which first brought on convulsion fits. She was uncertain how long these fits continued, but the first perception she had of returning sense was a most excruciating pain in her stomach. On a sudden this pain vanished, and her right arm was instantaneously flung into an involuntary and perpetual motion.

She had in vain made use of the most likely means to conquer her disorder; which, at the time she gave me this account, had continued without any abatement for upwards of sixteen months, nine of which she had been a patient in the Exeter Infirmary.

This motion of the arm was like the swing of a pendulum, which it resembled also in being regular and incessant. It was besides quick, and so strong, that the hand was at every vibration flung up higher than her head. And what adds much to this singular phenomenon is, that it neither fatigued her, nor abated her strength; yet if by any means whatever it was stopped, even though by herself, a most severe pain immediately seized her stomach, and convulsion fits were the certain consequence.

Once, at my request, she took a light walking cane in her hand, which she had no sooner done, but this motion becoming irregular and unequal, the pain of her stomach returned with extreme violence, and she fell into the strongest convulsion fit I ever saw; out of which she did not recover till the arm had, after infinite struggles, returned to its accustomed vibration.

With respect to the general state of her health, this patient was no ways disordered. Her appetite and digestion were good, the catamenia were regular, and the other secretions and evacuations were perfect. Her sleep, indeed, was too short; it seldom lasted longer than three or four hours. During sleep the motion of her arm ceased; but the instant she awoke (and she was always awakened by a pain of the stomach,) it returned, aud continued without intermission for the remainder of the four and twenty hours.

After she had drank the waters and bathed for about a month, finding no amendment in her complaint, I prescribed for her a medicine composed of assafætida and opium. She began by taking a grain of opium every day, and gradually increased the quantity to four grains a day. In the use of this remedy, together with bathing and drinking the waters, she persisted for another month; but without any kind of benefit. On the contrary, those days she went into the bath her spirits and strength were much weakened. She was ordered, therefore, to omit bathing, and to have her arm and the spine of her back pumped every or every other day, for as long a time as she could bear it. Drinking the waters and her medicine were continued; for I observed the opium neither occasioned drowsiness, relaxation of the solids, or any defect in the performance of those functions on which health depends.

It was near three weeks after she had commenced this last plan, before any alteration was made in her disorder; when as she was one day using the pump, the motion of her arm suddenly changed, and having been perpendicular became horizontal.

This change made it evident that a different set of muscles were now affected, on which account it was not unreasonable to suppose, that by persevering in those measures which had occasioned such an alteration, the entire cure of the disease might in time be effected. Nor did the supposition happen to be wrong; for this horizontal motion grew gradually less and less, till it entirely ceased, and the arm became obedient to her will. Before she left the Hospital, having remained in it six months, her arm was so perfectly restored to its natural motion and strength, that I have seen her carry with it a brass bucket full of water, and assist in washing the ward she belonged to.

Upon her discharge she went into service, but came back to us about two months afterwards. She had felt some slight attacks of pain in her stomach, and therefore dreaded the return of the involuntary motion of the arm. But by occasionally taking a few warm aloetic purges, and drinking the waters daily for about five or six weeks, (neither bathing nor pumping being necessary,) her stomach was set to rights, and the return of the spasm of her arm prevented.

ON CUTANEOUS DISEASES.

FROM the earliest periods the Bath waters have been celebrated as a most effectual remedy in cutaneous disorders; and although the classification of the different varieties of lepra, psoriasis, &c. were little attended to and less understood, yet experience had so clearly defined the different stages of these diseases benefited by the waters, that their misapplication was next to an impossibility. The medicinal virtues of these waters, it is reasonable to suppose, were first applied for the relief of those scurfy and scaly affections of the skin which, from a variety of causes, have tormented mankind from the creation of the world; and it is rather remarkable, that not only have the beneficial effects of the Bath waters been celebrated and brought into notice from accidental benefit in cutaneous disorders, but almost similar fabulous accounts have, with some varieties, stamped the benefit of most of the sulphureous waters and hot springs discovered on the continent.

Whatever may have been the foundation of the fame of the Bath waters in diseases of the skin, whether originating from the leprous King Bladud, or, as is much more probable, learnt from "sad experience," still their efficacy has been too long acknowledged to give the smallest handle to scepticism.

The varieties of lepra and the different species of psoriasis are the cutaneous affections most commonly sent to Bath for the benefit of the waters. The former is characterised by scaly patches of different sizes, but nearly of a circular form, affecting different parts of the body, and gradually extending. The scaly patches by accumulation form a thick prominent crust, which falling off is continually reproduced. This disease is not accompanied by much constitutional derangement, but is attended with troublesome itching, and often a watery discharge when the scales are detached. In severe cases the nails of the fingers and of the toes are much thickened, become altered in their colour, and incurvated at the extremities.

The psoriasis is likewise marked by a scaly state of the cuticle, of an irregular figure, and for the most part accompanied by fissures of the skin. This disease from its situation has different names assigned it by Dr. Willan, as the P. palmaria, P. labialis, P. scrotalis, &c. but the most obstinate variety is the Psoriasis inveterata, of which we shall give an account in Dr. Bateman's own words. "The psoriasis inveterata begins in separate irre-"gular patches, which extend and become con-"fluent, until at length they cover the whole "surface of the body, except a part of the face, or "sometimes the palms of the hands and soles of "the feet, with an universal scaliness, interspersed "with deep furrows, and a stiff, hard, and "thickened state of the skin. The production "of scales is so rapid, that large quantities are "found every morning in the patient's bed. The "nails become convex, thickened, and opaque, "and are frequently renewed; and at an advanced "period, especially in old people, extensive exco-"riations sometimes occur, with a discharge of "their lymph, followed by a hard dry cuticle, "which separates in large pieces. In this extreme "degree it approaches very closely to the invete-"rate degree of lepra vulgaris in all respects; the "only difference being in the form of the patches "before they coalesce."

The cause of these affections is often involved in great obscurity; many authors suppose them to originate from cold and moisture, others from particular kinds of food, and many from suppressed evacuations or hereditary predisposition. They are not considered contagious; and they affect both sexes, but generally about the middle period of life.

In all cases of lepra the diet should be light and moderate, malt liquor and spirits should be avoided. "A frequent use of the warm bath," observes Dr. Bateman, "with which a moderate degree "of friction may be combined, contributes to remove "the scales, and to soften the skin; or if the eruption be confined to the extremities, local ablution "may be sufficient." In more violent cases, however, local applications are necessary in conjunction with warm bathing; and Dr. Willan particularly recommends the tar ointment, or the nitrate ointment modified, according to the irritability of the skin, or the virulence of the eruption. Many internal remedies have been advised in these complaints; the arsenical solution, pitch pills, sulphur with soda or nitre, tinct. lyttæ, mercurial preparations, particularly the plummer's pill, and all these medicines with very little effect, excepting the last.

The plummer's pill taken internally, and the nitrate ointment externally applied, have, undoubtedly, been used with the greatest advantage; but many cases occur, where these remedies are very inefficient without the use of the Bath waters. The great advantage of bathing is evident from the disease occurring (if at all) at a much longer period, and in a much milder form.

It is to be lamented, that under the most successful management of cutaneous diseases they are apt to return; but in some very distressing cases which have come under my eye, and where the patients had been previously affected for many years with little intermission, a course of the Bath waters, both internal and external, has appeared to clear the skin, promote a proper perspiration, and renovate the constitution, and has enabled the patient on a return of the complaint easily to keep it under by having recourse to a modified preparation of the nitrate ointment.

This latter application will often appear at first to aggravate the complaint, occasioning great redness and irritation of the cuticle; this will, however, subside in a few days, and the advantage be more apparent in proportion to the irritation of the remedy.

The internal use of the waters is often of great service in psoriasis inveterata, where there is sometimes disordered state of the stomach; and the bowels should likewise be attended to previous to the exhibition of the waters.

I have not observed that the various species of scald head, or porrigo, are more relieved by the use of the Bath water than common warm water. The increased irritation occasioned by the collection of dry and furfuraceous eruption between the roots of the hair, require the constant use of soft soap and warm water prior to the use of the nitrate ointment, which is the only effectual remedy, and which, if properly persevered in, will always cure the complaint. Its failure nine times in ten depends on the remedies not being properly applied.

Another cuticular disease, very much benefited by the warm bathing, is the ichthyosis, or fish-skin disease. This disorder "is characterized by a "thickened, hard, rough, and, in some cases, "almost horny texture of the integuments of the "body, with some tendency to scaliness, but with-"out the deciduous exfoliations, the distinct and "partial patches, or the constitutional disorder "which belong to lepra and psoriasis. Patients "afflicted with ichthyosis are occasionally much "harassed with inflamed pustules, or with large "painful boils on different parts of the body; it "is also remarkable that they never seem to have "the least perspiration or moisture of the skin."

"When a portion of the hard scaly coating is "removed, it is not soon produced again. The "easiest mode of removing the scales is to pick "them off carefully with the nails, from any part "of the body, while it is immersed in hot water. "The layer of cuticle which remains after this "operation, is harsh and dry; and the skin did "not, in the cases that occurred, recover its usual "texture and softness, but the scales were pre-"vented from forming afterwards by the repeated "use of the warm bath, along with moderate "friction."

Pitch pills are strongly recommended by Dr. Bateman in many of these scaly eruptions; I have, however, never seen any benefit derived from them, though in some instances the patient has taken to the amount of nearly a hundred in a day.

The impetigo, ringworm, or tetter, and its varieties, are likewise much benefited by the use of the warm bath; and either the zinc ointment, or the nitrate very much lowered, should be applied afterwards. In short, in all these cutaneous affections the merits of our hot springs have been so long acknowledged, that a liberal benefactor formerly erected a bath solely for the use of leprous patients, and it still, with the common people, goes by the name of the leper's bath.

We shall now state the authorities who have celebrated the Bath waters in diseases of the skin. Dr. Pierce says, "I do know that for more than "forty years that I have lived here, there hath not "one past wherein there hath not been more than "a few instances of very great cure done upon "leprous, scabby, and scurfy persons; and more, "perhaps, might have been done, if they had bathed, "as Bladud did, in mud and water together. But "the nicety of our age is satisfied with nothing but "fresh baths; whereas in many cases (and this par-"ticularly) the mud is as effectual (if not more so) "than the purest of the water."

Dr. Charlton, after enumerating many Hospital cases, closes with the following observations:

" These diseases, 'tis presumed, will be thought " sufficient proofs of the efficacy of Bath waters in " diseases of the skin. But should further evi- " dence be required, the registers of the Hospital " will afford it. By them we find, that, from a " a period of thirteen years, 241 lepers had been " received into the house. Of this number 122 " were perfectly cleansed, 85 were much benefited, " 12 received no benefit, 4 died, 11 were improper " to be continued, and 7 were discharged for irre- " gularity. During the same period the Hospital " has admitted 50 patients under various sorts of " scorbutic eruptions; of these 26 were cured, 18 " were much relieved, one died, and 5 were im- " proper, from hectical symptoms, to make use of " the waters."

After alluding to the advantages of the waters in leprous cases, Dr. Falconer observes, " the use " of the bath, after a few times trial, generally " produces an abatement of the itching, and a " desquamation, in some degree, of the leprous " crusts, and of course renders the skin more soft " and pliable. This course is usually accompanied " with the use of the waters internally in moderate " quantities as about a pint daily, which are thought " to second the good effects of the bath, by pro- " moting a free and gentle perspiration."

Sir G. Gibbes recommends the waters strongly in these complaints. He says, "there is no disorder "in the cure of which the Bath waters have been "more celebrated than leprosy. This term com- "prehends in general a great variety of cutaneous "affections, it being indiscriminately applied to all "those eruptions of the skin which are scaly. "The Bath waters have appeared to me very ser- "viceable in cleansing the skin, and where the "cuticle was irritated in curing the disorder."

Whatever may be the mode in which these waters produce their beneficial effects, nothing is more certain, that in cutaneous eruptions, where the patient has been following the best advice for years, and where in many instances they have been deemed incurable at other hospitals, the waters here have produced the most wonderful effects, not only in removing the complaint for the present, but in preventing a return for a long period, and often removing it altogether.

The local applications we have already alluded to in aid of the waters, their mode of application, and strength, must be discretionally used according to the length of standing and virulence of the disease.

The cases we have brought forward are wholly Hospital cases, from Drs. Oliver and Charlton; and attention should be paid to the length of time required for the steady perseverance of the water in the removal of these distressing complaints, as it cannot be expected they can be relieved in a very short time, and without the most assiduous attention.

Sarah Collins, aged 28, of the parish of Hammersmith, about seven years ago got a surfeit by drinking cold water when she was very hot. This surfeit shewed itself in an eruption all over her breast, which was removed by a salivation in St. George's Hospital; since which operation she has never seen her menses. Upon returning to her work the humour shewed itself violently, and continues so to do; for the cure of which she has been advised by many eminent physicians and surgeons to try the Bath waters; and she having not wherewithal to subsist herself at Bath during the time necessary for obtaining a cure, she begs the benefit of your Hospital, for which she is judged a proper object. W. O.

Discharged cured, having been a patient 254 days.

We may learn from this case, that though a salivation will clear the skin from such eruptions for a time, yet that it doth not always free the constitution from the seeds of the disease; which, when the vessels begin to fill again, and the strength of the patient to return, will bud out afresh. It is scarcely, therefore, worth while to put a patient to the inconvenience of so troublesome a discipline for so uncertain and temporary an advantage; especially as mercurials internally given by way of alterative will often produce more lasting effects. For this patient was cured, together with drinking the waters and bathing, by taking pills night and morning, which were composed of the *pulvis plummeri* and *pil. rufi.*

Samuel Wingrove, aged 17 years, has been afflicted with a leprosy three years. He was bred to husbandry; being heated, and in a profuse sweat, by hay-making, he sat down upon the ground, and drank freely of cold small beer and cider. About an hour afterwards he grew sick and vomited, had a constant head-ache, and remained much out of order for a week; he then grew well enough to be able to work as usual. About a month afterwards a small red spot appeared just below his right elbow; it spread and itched violently; it grew moist, and the ichor which oozed from it soon concreted into a branny scurf, as white as snow. Spots of the same kind appeared soon afterwards in great numbers round the elbows, knees, hands, fingers, feet, and toes, and a few in his face. His body remained quite clear from any eruption. He said his mother was subject to the same disease on her skin, if she ever drank freely of cold liquors when she was hot.

His lips were often swoln; and when he heated himself by exercise, especially after walking and hanging down his arms, his hands would swell, and the blotches would burst, chap, and bleed; but they were soon covered with the white crust after rest, and the swellings decreased.

This youth was of a florid, healthy complexion, a good skin, and sanguine constitution. In December he was interrupted in his course of drinking and bathing by a cold, which required bleeding and other proper means to relieve it.

This distemper is generally attended with costiveness, which the waters rather increase. To prevent which he was forced to have frequent recourse to opening medicines during his whole course.

He was admitted July 3d, and was discharged clean, that is, free from eruptions, Jan. 10th, the year following.

Elizabeth Jordan, aged 16 years, of a florid, healthy complexion, and good skin. Two years ago she first perceived small red spots about her knees, which spread gradually, oozed a little limpid humour, which concreted into a white farinaceous crust, the scales of which were continually falling off, and as constantly succeeded by fresh ones. They afterwards appeared about the elbows, wrists, and the outside of her arms and legs; her body was quite free from any eruptions; the crust itched intolerably. She attributed her disease to her having drank large draughts of cold liquors when she had been much heated by violent exercise or hard labour.

She had menstruated once, about sixteen months before she came hither; but from that time she had never had the least shew till she was taken into the Hospital. After her first bathing the menses appeared, and she continued regular all the while she was in the house; but they kept the periods of three weeks.

She was taken into the London Hospital soon after the first appearance of the eruptions, where she continued ten weeks. She was then discharged *little better*. A month after she was re-admitted, and continued in the Hospital sixteen weeks, when she was discharged *much better*. But eruptions breaking out afresh, she was recommended to us.

Long before any eruption appeared, her feet used to chap and run every winter, and were so sore that she could not go or stand.

Her upper lip often swelled, as it usually does in scrofulous cases.

She was admitted May 20th, and was discharged clean January 10th following.

When she came in she was prepared by bleeding and purging, as she was of a full habit and sanguine complexion. Afterwards she drank the waters moderately, and bathed three times a week all the while she was in the house. The costiveness to which she was subject was prevented by a lenitive electuary, with sulphur.

Benjamin Orford, about fifteen years ago, got a surfeit (so the country people call any great sudden alteration of the blood and juices by drinking cold liquors when they are very hot.) From that time he always felt a weight at the pit of his stomach, attended with faintness and sickness. About six years ago he lay ill of a fever three weeks, in which he was bled and blistered. A fortnight after he recovered from the fever, a red spot, as big as a half-crown, appeared on his right arm, upon which there soon grew a white, thick, chapped crust, which sometimes bled. The next summer that disappeared; but towards the autumn the same kind of spots appeared in his legs, and on several other parts of his body. He was 30 years of age, of a sanguine complexion, and hardy make.

After bleeding and purging, he drank the waters, and bathed three times a week, except when he was interrupted in his course by some feverish disorders; which obliged him to omit bathing and drinking the waters, till, by evacuations and the saline draughts, with a proper regimen, he could again use them safely.

The crusts were all washed off, but the redness and itching remained. He was discharged June 14th, *much better.*

William Popjoy, aged 24 years. About two years ago he frequently indulged himself in large draughts of cold water and small beer, when he was heated by walking very fast; soon after he felt great sickness at his stomach, and pain in his head, which continued a fortnight. Then small pimples appeared about his wrist, with a sense of burning heat, and violent itching. Those pimples enlarged themselves into boils, which grew very painful, inflamed, and suppurated, discharging an ichorous matter, which hardened into a white scab, rugged, uneven at the edges, with a black speck in the middle. The base remained red, inflamed, and spreading every way, but unequally from the centre. In three or four days the scab dried, separated, and fell off; a fresh inflammation came on, a suppuration and crust followed as before. These eruptions appeared in every part of the body by turns, but chiefly in spring and autumn.

This man was a tiler by trade; his diet was chiefly coarse bread and cheese, and fat bacon.

In February he complained of a pain and coldness at the pit of his stomach, and in his bowels. It is very common for persons who are under cure for skin diseases to be troubled with such complaints, when the eruptions are removed by bathing. Sometimes they are seized with violent head-aches and nervous disorders;

but bleeding, a gentle purge, and then diaphoretic medicines, generally relieve them in a few days, and enable them to go on with bathing again, though it may not be proper to let them go into the water as frequently, or to stay in it as long as they used to do.

This man was discharged cured April 17th.

Joseph Porter, of Trowbridge, aged 23 years, was, about three months past, seized with an erysipelas, proceeding, as it is supposed, from an obstructed perspiration, occasioned by his being exposed to long journies in wet weather; which, by the use of medicines, became in a great measure subdued; but it has since returned at intervals, and at present seems inclined to a leprosy, but in all other respects he is healthy.

R. D.

This man had eruptions on many parts of his body, which appeared in small bladders, and being broke by scratching, or being rubbed by his shirt, discharged a little sharp watery matter: this soon concreted into a dry scab, which crumbled off, and left the part under it pretty sound. About three years ago he had been infected by an itch; which, after two months from its first appearance, had been cured by a black ointment, probably mercurial.

He was feverish several times while he was in the house, which obliged him to leave off the water and bathing, and to use evacuations and the saline draughts.

This kind of eruption, which owes its origin to an itch ill cured, we find to be very obstinate. This person drank the waters and bathed several months without much benefit, fresh eruptions breaking out as fast as the old ones were washed away. To assist the waters, therefore, he took two drachms of a solution of one grain of *mercurius sublimat. cor.* in two ounces of brandy, every morning for a fortnight. This medicine made him a little sick, but never vomited or purged him. It kept up a free perspiration, and increased the quantity of urine. It must not be continued too long. I have known it to bring on violent head-aches, and sometimes pains in the stomach and bowels. After he had done taking this solution he returned to bathing, which then perfected his cure; and he was discharged after being in the Hospital six months.

Thomas Hutchinson, of Taunton, about seven years ago had a cutaneous eruption that was thought to be the itch, and was treated as such, on which it disappeared; since that time it has made its appearance every spring and fall, but by anointing and taking alterative medicines, has often disappeared, till about Christmas last; then a dry scab appeared on his head, and since that on his face, and other parts of his body, which does not go off by the former treatment, and is now become the true furfuraceous leprosy. This is the true state of his case, as taken from himself.

F. A.

This man's complaint was much of the same nature with that of Joseph Porter.

At first the waters and bathing had very little effect; he therefore took the foregoing solution, after which bathing took place, and he was discharged cured, Sept. 19th, having been admitted June 9th, of the same year. His disorder was of seven years standing.

This is to certify, that Mary Clark, belonging to the parish of Blagdon, and now living in Axbridge, is about the age of 32, and labours under the following disorder. That ever since she can remember, she has been subject at spring and fall to have cutaneous eruptions, mostly like the itch, break out about her; that her father was always the same, but by taking (at the time of its appearance) a little gentle physic, it used to go off, till about ten years since she happened to strike her leg against a stone, and bruised it, whereupon it ulcerated, and was very painful; she applied to a great many pretenders to surgery, but in vain. She then was carried to Mr. Lucas, surgeon, at Wells, but in a miserable condition, with both legs and thighs very much tumified and inflamed; and when she rubbed it, (as she could not sometimes avoid, through the violent itching,) it would break out in small pustules, and discharge a thin glutinous matter; she had likewise, at the same time, branny-like scales upon her arm and both knees, and very often aching pains in her legs, thighs, and arms, especially at night, when warm in bed. She was seven weeks under Mr. Lucas's care at Wells; in which time she was (with taking medicines) made much better; but it was near twelvemonths before the disorder was seemingly conquered. Ever since, she breaks out as before at spring and fall; but not to that height, till about two months since, when it appeared all over her body like the itch. She was blooded, took physic, and anointed, which almost carried off the eruptions about her body, but settled it in her leg; and now she was in the same manner as when she first applied to Mr. Lucas, only that her thighs are not so much inflamed as they were then, but in every other particular much the same. She was married before she applied to Mr. Lucas, and her husband is since dead, but never had the appearance of any such disorder about him. Her child is five or six years old, and never had any symptoms of it till his mother's late illness, when it came on in the same sort of itching eruptions. It is observed, that the woman and her parents always had the character of virtuous people. W. B.

The mother and child were both admitted, and both discharged cured. Patients 265 days.

This is a history of a violent scorbutic humour, which is not unworthy attention. It must be observed, that the husband, who lay in the same bed with his wife, was not infected; as likewise that the child shewed no signs of having such a disorder in its constitution till it arrived at the fifth or sixth, I should rather think the seventh, year of its age, at which period all the fluids undergo a new fermentation, and the circulation becomes strong enough to separate such humours from the blood, and to expel them through the skin.

Many *private* cases might be adduced in support of the benefit derived from the Bath Waters in these cutaneous disorders, as the guides at the baths can amply testify. Independent, however, of the unpleasant feeling attached to such publicity, the above recorded facts will sufficiently demonstrate their utility in this distressing and loathsome class of diseases.

Notwithstanding we have endeavoured to give a full account of the principal maladies which are benefited by the Bath Waters, yet there are many other affections, although not particularly indicated, that in certain stages receive the greatest benefit from their use. Thus gravelly concretions are very much assisted in their passage by using the warm bath, as most gouty patients can testify, gravel being the constant companion of gout. Whenever, therefore, a patient suspects, from pains about the kidnies, or irritation about the neck of the bladder, that a concretion of gravelly matter is endeavouring to force a passage, he should immediately go into the warm bath, and remain there forty or fifty minutes, or as long as possible without fainting, nothing contributing so effectually to assist the expulsion of the calculus, either from the urinary passages or from the biliary ducts.

The old authors recommended very large quantities of the Bath water to be taken inwardly for these attacks. If it proved of service, it must have been from its quantity, as it could not exercise any specific action on the gravel. If, however, as Dr. Falconer and Sir G. Gibbes suppose, the Bath waters have a diuretic property independent of their bulk and heat, quarts and gallons would materially encourage this determination, and of course assist the passage of the calculus. The bathing in these cases should never be neglected; and is most strongly recommended by Hippocrates, in the following passage, "*Quod si calculorum* "*dolor intolerabiliter affligit, in aquam calidam* "*te dimitte. Veruntamen ne ipsa, sicut paulo* "*ante ostendimus, abutare; nam calida perfusio* "*dolorem mitigat quidem, sed vires etiam exsol-* "*vit, quæ morbi causam et quicquid in corpore* "*inutile est, discutiunt.*"

In long habitual cases of diarrhæa I have witnessed the most essential benefit from the Bath waters, both drinking and bathing, and should certainly recommend a trial where other remedies have failed. It often happens, however, that these distressing cases of long continuance are very much connected with biliary derangement, and prior to the use of the waters, a dose of calomel and rhubarb should be administered to give them every chance of success.

The bowels in these cases should be kept warm, and in obstinate dysenteric affections a wide flannel roller swathed round the whole of the bowels has been of most decided service.

In dropsical cases the waters have also been advised, particularly by the late Dr. Lysons; at the present day they are not much relied upon, neither have I seen them administered in these disorders with any advantage.

Œdematous swellings are very much relieved by the waters ; and when the bathing is assisted with gentle friction, it is particularly serviceable, by increasing the action of the absorbent vessels. Their internal use will also strengthen the stomach and constitution, and with other means tend to correct the disposition to œdema.

In all scrophulous tumours, glandular or mesenteric affections, they may be used with the greatest advantage. In these formidable complaints, however, they can only be considered as powerful auxiliaries, and other remedies must be united to work that change in the constitution, without which no permanent benefit can be expected. Although the sea water has been considered a specific in scrofulous and glandular tumours, yet experience has fully proved how inadequate that remedy is for the removal of these complaints; and the number of disappointments which constantly occur have materially diminished our faith in salt water and sea bathing.

Whatever may be the advantage of sea bathing, I am convinced much more benefit is likely to be derived from a steady perseverance in the use of our warm baths, aided by mercurial, antimonial, or tonic remedies, according to the age of the patient, and stage of this Proteus disease.

The remedy I have principally advised, in union with the bath, (independent of occasional purgatives,) has been a combination of bark and burnt sponge; which, if persevered in a sufficient length of time, generally succeeds in restoring the tone of the vessels, and promoting the absorption of the lymphatic glands. In very considerable scrofulous enlargements, repeated blisters or stimulating embrocations have been of great service, by exciting the absorbents to a more vigorous action.

The enlargement of the lymphatic glands will in many cases, arise from debility alone, without the suspicion of scrofulous or hereditary taint; and it is in cases of this kind, as arising solely from debility, that the sea air is of service, acting as a tonic by bracing the constitution. Not that in every case of scrofula there is any specific in sea air or sea bathing; for Dr. Hamilton, in his Observations on Scrofula, expressly points out, that if sea water and air were specifics, scrofulous diseases would be unknown in seaport towns, but so far from that being the case, he is inclined to think the disease there "is really more severe and "distressing."*

Where children labour under enlargement of the mesenteric glands, and emaciation, loss of strength, and confined hard bowels are the consequence, the warm bathing will very materially assist the other

* Hamilton on Scrofula, p. 161.

remedies which may be advised; and with the use of gentle friction to the abdomen, will promote the action of the lymphatic system, and thus aid in removing the induration of the glands.

These glandular obstructions are often productive of that disease so distressing to children, and so difficult, in some instances, to remove,—termed the rickets. The general debility, tumid, hard belly, costive bowels, and enlarged joints,* which in a great measure constitute this disease, are much more relieved by the assistance of warm bathing than the employment of the cold bath, which has been generally recommended. If with the use of the warm bath are combined tonics, as bark or steel, with the occasional use of purgatives, a nutritive diet, moderate exercise, and pure air, relief will be certain, if the disorder arise from debility only; but if the complaint has its origin in a scrofulous disposition or hereditary taint, the success must be very doubtful. By recommending warm bathing in preference to the cold we do not mean to decry the utility of the latter; but every one must have seen instances where the debility has been too much to allow of the shock experienced from cold bathing; and under these circumstances it has done harm. Where, however, the child, by the use of tonics

* The bones become soft and cartilaginous, exhibiting throughout an aerolated structure, the cells containing a gelatinous substance. Bichat thinks that, as well as a diseased state of the cellular structure of the bone, the periosteum is thickened.

and warm bathing, has in some degree recovered from the general debility, the cold bathing afterwards may be resorted to with great advantage.

After all, the disease of rickets very often depends on the state of the bowels; and constant purgatives, with now and then a slight mercurial dose, will relieve the disease much more effectually than all the tonics. Whenever, therefore, the belly becomes hard, the spirits flag, and the appetite diminishes, these indications point out the necessity of attention to the alimentary canal.

In all accidental lamenesses, whether arising from falls, strains, or bruises, when the inflammation has subsided, and nothing but the debility remains, the greatest advantage is derived from pumping. Likewise in bursal swellings, and contractions, pains, and rigidity from fractured limbs, both bathing and pumping will be found eminently serviceable.

Many cases have been related by authors, where the bathing has been particularly useful in promoting conception; and formerly the ostensible object with many ladies in coming to Bath was with this expectation. There is no doubt it has a very salutary effect in cases of this description; also, when from frequent miscarriages there has been great consequent debility of the uterus. Many instances of this beneficial effect are related by Guidot, Pierce, and Oliver; but the circumstance which in former days fully established their credit as a prolific remedy, was the successful bathing of the unfortunate consort of James II.

Having brought the subject of the Bath Waters to a conclusion, we trust, that whatever errors may be committed in the execution, still the intent may plead in mitigation, and that the facts brought forward will evince to the candid reader, that the Bath Waters are neither an insignificant nor an inefficient remedy; and that their effects require only to be known to be duly appreciated.

The principal object in the progress of this work has been, to support the credit of the Waters on the basis of practical experience, devoid of all theoretical speculation; and certainly they need no elaborate encomium, when their merits are carefully examined on this broad foundation. When used with those precautions it has been our study to suggest, these healing springs will be most deservedly ranked as one of the greatest blessings and benefits conferred on this happy island; and may be truly denominated the real Pool of Bethesda.

THE GENERAL HOSPITAL.

THIS noble Hospital, from the records of which we have so largely extracted, and which will continue an everlasting monument of the salutary effects of the Bath Waters, was founded in the year 1738, opened for the reception of patients in the year 1742, and is calculated to admit 133 patients, provided the generous benefactions of the public contribute an income sufficient to support this number.

This building was originally designed for the purpose of extending the benefit of the Bath waters to every part of the kingdom; consequently none but strangers are admissible, and their cases must be approved by the Medical Committee, as coming within the range of diseases benefited by the Bath waters.

It was very properly considered, that there are many institutions in this charitable city, where the poor inhabitants may apply for relief, and have every advantage of the waters gratuitously, by application to the proper authorities.

At present this charity is supported partly by the income of its own fund, partly by its annual subscribers, occasional donations, and collections made twice a year at the different churches in Bath, in which charity sermons are preached for that purpose.

For the information of those subscribers who may wish to recommend patients for admission, we subjoin the regulations of the Hospital; and for the direction of those who wish to remember this institution in their last will, we shall likewise give the testamentary form.

CONDITIONS OF ADMISSION INTO THE GENERAL HOSPITAL AT BATH.

1. The case of the patient must be described by some physician or person of skill in the neighbourhood of the place where the patient has resided for some time; and this description must be sent in a letter, (franked or post-paid,) directed to the Register of the General Hospital at Bath.

The age and name of the patient must be mentioned in the description of the case; and the persons who describe it are desired to be particular in the enumeration of the symptoms; so that neither improper cases may be admitted, nor proper ones rejected, by the physicians and surgeons, who always examine and sign the cases as proper or improper, previous to their being laid before the Weekly Committee.

If the patient has any fever upon him, as long as the fever continues he will be deemed improper —Patients with coughs, attended with pain in the chest or spitting of blood, are improper; as are also those with abscesses, or with any external ulcers, until such ulcers are healed.

From want of attention to the above particulars, very imperfect descriptions of cases have been, and are still, sent; and many patients have been discharged as improper soon after their admission, to the disappointment of the patients thus sent.

2. After the patient's case has been thus described, sent, and approved of as above, he must remain in his usual place of residence till he has notice of a vacancy, signified by a letter from the Register, accompanied with a blank certificate.

3. Upon the receipt of such a letter, the patient must set forward for Bath, bringing with him this letter, the parish certificate duly executed by the Minister and Parish Officers where such patient is legally settled, and attested before two Justices for the county or city to which the patient belongs, and three pounds caution money if from any part of England or Wales; but if the patient come from Scotland or Ireland, then the caution money to be deposited before admission is the sum of five pounds.

4. Soldiers may, instead of parish certificates, bring a certificate from their Commanding Officers, signifying to what corps they belong, and that they shall be received into the same corps when discharged from the Hospital, in whatever condition they are. And the same is expected from the Governors of Chelsea and Greenwich Hospitals respecting their pensioners. But it is necessary that their cases be described, and sent previously, and that they bring with them three pounds caution money.

The intention of the caution-money is to defray the expenses of returning the patients after they are discharged from the Hospital, or of their burial in case they die there. The remainder of the caution-money, after these expenses are defrayed, will be returned to the person who deposited it.

All persons coming to Bath, under pretence of getting into the Hospital without having their cases thus described and sent previously, and leave given to come, will be treated as vagrants, as the Act of Parliament for the regulation of the Hospital requires.

N. B. If any patient should have the small-pox here, such person must be removed out of the House, and the caution-money defray the expenses thereof. Likewise, all persons who shall come into the Hospital, without decent and necessary apparel, must have such necessaries provided out of the said caution-money.

Persons who are pleased to favour this charity are desired to pay their charitable contributions into the hands of Messrs. Hoare and Co. bankers, London; or to the Treasurers at Bath, viz. Charles Phillott, esq; Sir William Watson, or Wyndham Goodden, esq; or may put their several contributions into the box placed in the Pump-Room, or into that in the Hospital, for that purpose.

Such as choose to be benefactors by their last will, have the following form recommended to them: "*Item*, I give and bequeath unto "A. B. and C. D. the sum of —— upon trust, and to the intent that "they, or either of them, do pay the same to the Treasurers for the time "being of the Hospital or Infirmary at Bath; which said sum of —— "I desire may be applied towards carrying on the charitable designs "of the Governors of that Hospital."

INDEX.

Printed by Richard Cruttwell,
St. James's-Street, Bath.